D0469849

Civic Center

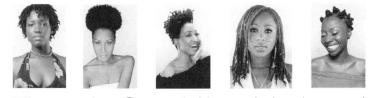

Thank God I'm Natural

The Ultimate Guide to Caring for and Maintaining Natural Hair

by: *Chris-Tia E. Donaldson*

Thank God I'm Natural -- The Ultimate Guide to Caring for and Maintaining Natural Hair
By Chris-Tia Donaldson
TgiNesis Press

Published in the United States by TgiNesis Press
Copyright © 2008 by Chris-Tia Donaldson

Publisher's Cataloging-In-Publication Data
(Prepared by The Donohue Group, Inc.)

Donaldson, Chris-Tia.
  Thank God I'm Natural : The Ultimate Guide to Caring for and Maintaining Natural Hair / Chris-Tia Donaldson.

  p. : ill. ; cm.

  Includes bibliographical references.
  ISBN: 978-0-9820944-0-2

1. Hairdressing of Blacks. 2. Hairstyles. 3. Hair--Care and hygiene. I. Title.

TT972 .D66 2008
646.7/24/08996073

Table of Contents

Acknowledgements

Although only one author's name appears on the cover of this book, it took a team of dedicated and talented people to pull a project like this together. I am delighted to have worked with these contributors -- and also honored to have the privilege of thanking them here.

First and foremost, I want to thank God for giving me the strength and courage to tell my story. I now see the meaning of it all and thank you for opening doors and creating opportunities that I never thought were possible.

I would also like to thank my family for always being there for me. Special gratitude to my parents for teaching me, from a young age, that I could do anything -- and for making so many sacrifices on my behalf. Mom and Dad, if it weren't for you, I would not be where I am today.

To Cuz, you are truly the wind beneath my wings. Thank you for your never-ending support and encouragement -- and for reading the first draft of every single chapter, even when they were long (and hopefully not too painfully boring). We've been through so much together and you will always mean the world to me.

To Anthony, Lord what can I say? When I met you for the first time at Starbucks, I had absolutely no hope of ever finishing this project. Thanks for all the text messages, phone calls and gmail chats. Your support and encouragement were invaluable and the only reason why I was able to keep that pen moving. I would have never found my *"voice"* without you.

To my editors, who were more than a major part of this book. In no particular order – Lawrence, Rebecca, Cassie, Danice, Leea, Kristy, Victoria, Ewurama, Nehezi, Zak, Charisse, Jaunqiue, Tonya, Dat Chick, Susan, Ellen, and Brett. Thanks for your unwavering dedication and for giving me your honest and constructive feedback.

Finally, to all of the women and men who agreed to be interviewed for this book and for believing in my cause. Your stories and experiences were an invaluable resource and inspiration.

If there is anyone I have left out, please forgive me but know that I am eternally grateful for your support and encouragement.

Chris-Tia Donaldson

Foreword

When I launched my website devoted to natural hair care in 2001, there was no roadmap for those of us bravely choosing to embark upon this fantastic journey. Back then, you basically considered yourself lucky if *Essence* featured Jill Scott on the cover rocking an Afro and a few tips for dealing with curly hair on the pages inside. The so-called "natural" magazines were also of very little help. Many of the styles showcased therein were expensive illusions, mostly created using extensions. These publications offered very little in the way of practical advice for women caring for their natural hair at home. Other than a few books here and there, those of us that wanted to go natural were pretty much left to our own devices when it came to taking care of our kinky tresses.

At first, I felt alone and discouraged. However, no sooner than I could say the words "Afro puffs," I was receiving close to fifty emails a day from women thanking me for the few digi-pics I posted in my online journal, showing my natural hair's progress. Today, www.MotownGirl.com is a place where women of color come to find love and support for their decision to wear their hair natural -- as well as step-by-step styling instructions, product reviews, and homemade hair care recipes. If only *Thank God I'm Natural* had been around back when I began my journey, what a difference it would have made!

The good news is that the interest in natural hair is now stronger than ever. Women continue to bid farewell to breakage, thinning edges, and hair loss caused by chemical straighteners. Unfortunately, a host of myths and misconceptions about our natural hair still abound. This is what makes *Thank God I'm Natural* so timely and unique. This book goes beyond the basics and takes the mystery out of caring for our hair in its natural state. It is also a wonderful resource, whether you're contemplating going natural or have already made the bold yet liberating conversion to this style.

Thank God I'm Natural reminds us (what we are so often in danger of forgetting) *that all healthy hair -- whether straight, nappy, kinky or coily – is good hair*. Whether you know Chris-Tia personally or end up getting to know her in the next few chapters, you'll soon see that she loves what she does and her passion shows on every single page. So, dive into your natural journey knowing that you have finally found the comprehensive guide you need to truly embrace your curly tresses. And whatever you do, enjoy every moment developing your own natural look -- and don't forget to send us pictures!

Alisha a.k.a "MotownGirl"

Introduction

I grew up in the 1980's -- before *"healthy"* was in and Whole Foods Supermarkets, Aquafina bottled water, and the Subway diet were all the rage. Back then, no one really cared or thought about the potential dangers of using chemical relaxers. We had no reason to be afraid, since we had no clue about the harm we were inflicting on ourselves by using these products.

So today, in this enlightened age, very few people believe me when I tell them I got my first perm when I was just four years old! My mom, like most black women, didn't know the first thing about caring for her daughter's hair -- let alone her own, in its natural state. When her stylist learned that I was tender-headed *(meaning - I screamed my head off at the mere sight of a rat-tail comb)*, she offered an easy solution; we would fix the *"problem"* with a relaxer. This moment marked the beginning of my love affair with chemical straighteners. For the next twenty-odd years, I would perm my hair religiously and spend literally thousands of dollars on trips to the salon and on products that promised longer, stronger, and healthier hair. And for what? All to counteract the damage and breakage caused by relaxers. So much for that easy solution…

1

Despite the fact that so much information is now available, it saddens me that we continue to *fix* our daughters' hair with a steady stream of dangerous chemicals. We often go to extreme lengths to protect our children from the solutions and chemical cocktails so dangerously lurking under the kitchen sink -- yet we turn around and apply these same toxic agents to their hair and scalps without ever questioning the impact on their health and safety!

On a deeper level, our sense of self worth is also jeopardized. By straightening our hair and our daughters' hair, we start to develop a subconscious belief at a very early age that something is inherently wrong with our kinky tresses. Some of us have even reached the point where we feel like we have no other option. Well, I am here to tell you, there *is* a better way. Even if you've been using relaxers for most of your life and don't know the first thing about caring for your hair naturally, know this: it can be done.

When I went natural in 2002, I had a million questions and, frankly, nowhere to turn for answers. At times, I felt extremely discouraged and overwhelmed by the lack of information at my disposal. But what started out as a simple quest for answers has become a full-blown passion of mine. I've met and talked with hundreds of women, from all walks of life. Although their reasons for going natural vary, women with kinky hair are fed up with the breakage and damage caused by relaxers. We're tried of watching our hairlines disappear and trying to hide our bald spots under wigs, weaves, and extensions. We're fed up with letting our tresses get in the way of intimate encounters and spending our entire Saturday mornings sitting in a beauty salon. We have better things to do with our time, like figuring out how to balance the demands of work and family. Finally, some of us just can't stand the thought of helping the manufacturers of these dangerous products get rich, preying on our insecurities.

So, this book is for you: women who are looking for change and new beginnings with their hair and their life in general. The hair care maintenance program found in this publication has been drawn from celebrity stylists' recommendations and firsthand accounts of women who have successfully made the transition from relaxed to natural hair. Filled with practical tips, *Thank God I'm Natural* will help you assess your hair type and give you the knowledge and tools you need to develop an effective hair care regimen and maintenance plan that will suit you for many years to come. You'll also find answers to some of the most frequently asked questions, product recommendations for your hair type, and photographs of women with different hair textures rocking the latest natural styles.

My ultimate goal in writing this book is to help you make your transition from relaxed to natural hair go as smoothly as possible. It's also meant to be a source of comfort and support during some of your difficult moments. When you feel alone or like giving up, flip through these pages and know that many women's lives have changed for the better once they let go of the chemicals and finally put an end to their hair abuse. See these women as a true inspiration and let them offer you proof that a change is both possible and necessary.

Again, welcome to your natural hair journey! Now that you've picked up this book, you're already well on your way to to achieiving that glorious crown that you've always dreamed of.

3

Chapter 1
My Story

IT WAS SATURDAY NIGHT and my place was *packed*!!! As *This Christmas* played loudly in the background, I could finally breathe a sigh of relief -- knowing that for once everything was going exactly according to plan. This year, I decided to make things easy on myself. Instead of doing all of the cooking as usual, I simply picked up a shrimp platter, a veggie tray, and a few desserts from Costco's. A quick and easy fix for what would otherwise have been several grueling hours of prepping, simmering, baking and roasting. All I had to do was take the teriyaki wings out of the oven and then everything would be set. What could be simpler, right? Wrong!

No amount of planning or preparation could have prepared me for what happened next. As I bent down and leaned my head towards the broiler, I could feel 475° of intense heat suddenly sweep across my face. My mouth opened in horror and my festive spirit was instantly transformed into disbelief when I realized that my wig's soft, flowing bangs had morphed into hard, melted plastic. It didn't take long for the unmistakable stench of burnt hair to permeate throughout my entire apartment and overpower the smell of everything -- even the sweet aroma of my Glade Christmas-Cookie plug-ins! There I stood, melted plastic bangs glued to my shiny, sweaty forehead -- and my friends waiting in the very next room . . . still hungry.

I knew from experience not to use curling irons on synthetic hair -- but the warning label on my wig said nothing about the danger of retrieving appetizers from the oven. I tried my best to pull it together and discreetly survey the damage, while at the same time thinking WWMD -- What Would Martha (Stewart) Do? After a moment or two of inspection, I determined the situation was hopeless. No amount of water, Ultra Sheen, or braid spray would ever bring my bangs back to life. It was a wrap, a goner. My wig was officially dead on arrival.

Fortunately, not all was lost; I had a back up plan. Unbeknownst to my family, friends, and co-workers, I'd been wearing wigs for close to two years -- ever since I graduated from law school – and now I had over thirty different styles in my collection. There were wigs for every occasion; short wigs, long wigs, red wigs, blonde wigs, kinky wigs, curly wigs, flip wigs, wavy wigs, and wiggy wigs. You name it -- I had it. Some girls collect shoes . . . I collected wigs.

Yes, I could look like Beyonce, Ashanti, or any girl in a rap video for a mere $24.99. But with that terrific flexibility and variety came a hefty price -- paranoia. What if my wig was on crooked or if, heaven forbid, a mighty gust of Chicago wind came and carried my precious hairpiece right down Michigan Avenue? Even worse was wearing a wig while dating! Let me tell you, while I had mastered the art of keeping men's hands out of *"my hair"*, it was a constant challenge (and emotionally quite stressful) to maintain my dirty little secret. Extensions are one thing to most men -- but wearing a wig involved a whole new layer of deception that inevitably lead to the *"Honey, there is something I have to tell you. This isn't my hair..."* conversation.

* * * *

IN RETROSPECT, I HAVE come to realize that most of my issues having to do with hair stems from the fact that I went to an all-white school for most of my childhood. You see, my parents were a product of the Civil Rights Era and made huge sacrifices to send me to a small private school for gifted children where I was fortunate enough to receive a first-rate education. There was just one problem: **For seven years, I was the ONLY black girl in my entire class.**

I had no problem fitting in socially with my white classmates. Yet, sometimes my kinky hair made me feel like a complete and total outsider. It was one thing to grow up watching white sitcoms from the 1980's like *The Wonder Years, Family Ties, and Growing Pains* -- but it's another story to go to school every day and be surrounded by a sea of white girls with flowing hair that hung down their backs. In contrast to their beautiful, blond, shimmering tresses, my short, brown hair seemed so dull and ugly.

To make matters worse, my cornrows with aluminum foil and colored beads on the ends made me stick out like a sore thumb. At this point, no one had seen or even heard of Venus and Serena Williams -- so there was no way I could possibly play this "ethnic" style off as cool. My cornrows were convenient and kept me from fussing with my hair. But everyday, I secretly prayed for long blond tresses that I could squirt pink L.A. gel in and pull back into a scrunchie.

I survived all this, of course -- but I was deeply impacted and emotionally scarred for years to come. This longing to physically blend in with my white female classmates coupled with a persistent feeling of dissatisfaction with my own appearance would prove to be the beginning of a decade-long battle with my hair, and my coming to grips with who I was a black woman.

* * * *

AFTER SEVEN YEARS AND countless hours of fretting over my kinky mane, I found diversity at last at Mercy High School for Girls. Although I was just one of forty black girls in a class of two hundred, I could show up with finger waves, a French roll, crimps, or all of the above -- and nobody ever asked questions like: *"Why don't you ever wear your hair down?"*, *"Why don't you wash your hair everyday?"*, or *"How do you get your hair to do that?"*

7

I had finally learned to accept my hair for what it was. Still, thanks to my experiences in elementary school, I continued to nurture an unhealthy obsession with growing my hair long. Like most black teenage girls, I preferred long, stringy hair that rested on my shoulders to a short, healthy, chin-length bob. In my efforts to achieve this seemingly unattainable measure of beauty, I tried every product on the market that promised to grow my hair -- from *Super Gro*, to *Doo Grow*, to *You Grow*. In the end, much to my own dissatisfaction, nothing really seemed to work. Most of the time, these products just left me with limp hair, a terribly greasy scalp, and bitter disappointment.

Despite the fact that my hair was now in the hands of a licensed professional, it still wasn't getting any longer. Unfortunately, my stylist's idea of healthy hair and mine were vastly different. Whenever my hair did grow, my beautician would relax my new growth within minutes of it sprouting from my scalp and then turn around and cut two inches off my ends. I fought long and hard to break this vicious cycle, but no matter how much money I spent or what products I used, I was always left sitting in the revolving leather salon chair, staring in the mirror at the inevitable, much hated chin-length bob.

* * * *

UPON GRADUTING FROM HIGH SCHOOL, I set off to Harvard for college. After careful consideration, I opted for a short pixie cut (think Halle Berry). It was a cute, stylish and extremely convenient. Most importantly, it was healthy. As I prepared for my journey somewhat content with my choice of hairstyle, it occurred to me that black salons would possibly be few and far between in the pretentious, lily-white Boston area. I had no choice but to prepare for the worst. When I stepped foot on campus, I arrived armed with a stove iron, a sit-under hair dryer, and a 1200-watt blow dryer. My friends often joked that they didn't know whether I was going to school to be a lawyer or a cosmetologist.

Little did I know that during this expedition I would be fortunate enough to find William – the talented, creative, magician of a hair dresser who I would eventually come to recognize as my very own personal hair God. Not only was he fierce when it came to laying it down style-wise, but he also specialized in healthy hair. As fate would have it, William was also the first person to ever suggest that I didn't need a perm.

I had very little success with relaxers up until this point -- so I decided to take his advice and start pressing my hair instead. After a few months, I noticed a considerable difference. My hair was now past my shoulders and in its healthiest condition ever. It was thick, full, and had *tons* of body. To my surprise, it was also growing because it wasn't constantly breaking off due to the damage from all the chemicals I had used so often before.

As happy as I was to finally achieve hair 'normalcy', the time and money necessary to maintain my locks was simply outrageous. I was making real progress -- but I was also spending over $50 a week – more than half my work-study pay check -- on a press and curl. I tried in vain not to get my hopes up and my heart set on having long, healthy hair only to have it break off again. All it would take was one bad relaxer, one bad dye job, or one bad haircut -- and I would be right back to where I started with the oh-so-dreaded chin length bob. It was a vicious, never-ending cycle. Something had to give.

After twenty-odd years of spending thousands of dollars to maintain my hair in tip-top condition -- scheduling exercise, vacations, and dates around my hair appointments (and often sitting in the beauty salon for five grueling hours on Saturday mornings) I had finally reached my breaking point. If I didn't want to spend the rest of my life consumed by my mane, I had no choice but to go natural. There was only one problem: I hadn't seen my natural texture in over twenty years.

* * * *

IN MY FINAL SEMESTER OF LAW SCHOOL, I made the transition to natural hair, wearing braids. With braids, there was no such thing as a bad hair day and I enjoyed the perk of not having to wake up forty-five minutes early just to curl my hair.

Better yet, when I took my braids down for the first time, I was amazed that my hair had grown nearly two inches. However, as luck would have it, on the eve of my newfound success, disaster would strike once again. Who knew it was necessary to detangle natural hair before taking a shower? Whoops! When the water hit my hair, my mane was *9* instantly transformed into a matted nest of knots and tangles. No amount of conditioner or oil sheen could ever reverse the damage, leaving me with no choice but to cut off **all** my hair. . . . **Three days later, I bought my first wig.**

Although it took some getting used to, at first, wearing a wig seemed like a very reasonable resolution to my hair dilemma. It was considerably less expensive and time consuming than having to constantly style my own hair and, by corporate America's standards, it was perfectly acceptable for the workplace. I eventually convinced myself that by wearing a wig, I had found the answer to my seemingly life-long hair struggles. At the time I didn't realize it, but it wouldn't be long until the false sense of security I had worked so hard to build up came crumbling down – right over the top of my chicken teriyaki.

* * * *

SEEING MY CHARRED WIG lying on the dresser the night of my holiday party was all it took for me to embrace my natural hair, once and for all. As I searched through my closet frantically looking for a suitable replacement -- I sat down amidst the strewn clothes, shoes and hair pieces, and broke down in tears. Then, it hit me: I was happy wearing hair in every color, texture, and length – but not my own.

Despite my overwhelming success in school and other areas of my life up to that point, I was deeply unhappy and still uncomfortable in my own skin. To top it off, I was teetering on the verge of getting fired from my first job fresh out of law school. My negative perceptions of my hair and its diminishing effect on my appearance in general left me less than confident at a time in my life when confidence was more critical than ever.

Deep down inside, I was miserable. After accepting a position at one of the top law firms in the nation straight out of law school, I once again felt major pressure to blend in with my white colleagues. I was working long hours and felt like I needed to be a younger version of the ultra beautiful, super smart, and sophisticated Claire Huxtable (from "*The Cosby Show*") in order to truly be accepted by my white co-workers.

10

Had I been practicing law for fifteen years and gained a strong reputation by this point, I might have felt more at ease with my decision to wear my hair natural. Unfortunately, there were only two black women in my department and I was one of them. I wasn't exactly looking to complicate matters by putting on my dashiki and rocking Bantu knots to my first client meeting.

I knew I needed to let go and stop wearing a wig -- but after two years of waking up every morning and putting one on, I couldn't stand the sight of myself without my synthetic tresses. Day in and day out, I would constantly make excuses to myself as to why I couldn't wear my natural hair uncovered. *My hair isn't long enough. I don't know what products to use. It only takes me five minutes to get ready in the morning. My colleagues would talk about me. My boyfriend would dump me. No one would ever find me attractive.*

To make matters worse, I had gotten used to having long silky, straight hair -- which drew compliments daily. When I wore a wig, it seemed as if I couldn't walk down the street without men telling me how much they loved my beautiful hair or women asking me who my stylist was. But behind my smile, I knew that it was all a lie and I lived in fear daily that the terrible truth would be discovered. I knew that something had to change, I simply did not have the confidence nor the courage to break free from this all-consuming crutch.

* * * *

I'M NOT GOING TO LIE: giving up my wig and wearing my hair completely natural was one of the single most difficult decisions I have ever made. After getting a perm for twenty-plus years, I didn't know the first thing about caring for my natural texture. I had no clue what products or styling tools to use or how to work with the tight, spongy curls sitting atop my head. Learning to do my hair was like teaching myself Swahili. I simply didn't know where to begin.

Then there was the issue of seeing the reactions of my friends and co-workers who would now know that I had been wearing some kind of extensions for the past two years. While my hair had grown quite long, *11* it wasn't silky or straight. Instead, it looked dry and dull -- like week-old cotton candy, because I had kept it covered for so long.

In addition to my apprehension over my dramatic change in appearance and the styling difficulties that came along with it, for the first time in my life, I also had to deal with the daily challenge of seeking a new job after my boss informed me that my work fell quite short of meeting my department's expectations. Needless to say, wearing a wig had taken a major toll on my self-esteem, and was affecting me on many levels, both personally and professionally.

Ironic, isn't it? It turned out that wearing a wig had made very little difference after all -- and hadn't spared me from being told that I didn't have a future with my firm. After putting so much time and effort into appeasing my conservative white colleagues, it hadn't truly helped or changed anything.

In hindsight, I should have pulled a Jill Scott or Erykah Badu on my very first day at my law firm and spent the countless hours I had invested worrying about my appearance into focusing on my job performance. If only I had known and appreciated then how truly beautiful my own, natural hair is – it would have saved me so much heartache, expense, and wasted energy. I walked away from the firm with my pride wounded, however, much more importantly, with the realization that my own lack of confidence and esteem lay at the heart of my failure. This truth was much more painful than the simple disappointment of coming close to being fired.

After several months of working tirelessly to find a new position, God stepped in and blessed me with a new job, where I felt like I could not only be myself, but that I also had the potential to become a tremendous asset to the firm's already outstanding talent. After gladly accepting the job, I was amazed at how comfortable I was with my decision to wear my hair natural on the very first day.

Surprisingly enough, I was given more opportunities and received better mentoring than I did at my first firm. Due to the change in professional atmosphere, I was finally able to prove my talent and dedication to my work. This was a welcome change from my first law firm, where I fought so desperately to accommodate society's unattainable beauty standard for black women (and not my own).

It was such a refreshing feeling to be able to work at a place where I could be myself and wear my own, natural hair -- without thinking or worrying about how I would be perceived. I grew more comfortable daily, and for the first time ever, I didn't hesitate to come to work with my hair pulled back into a puff, braids, or two strand twists. The quality of my work was praised and my performance was never questioned (since I could now focus on what was really important, my work – and not my hair).

I was beginning to realize how silly and unnecessary my concerns had been before. The more I loved and accepted my natural hair, the more people applauded my work and complimented me. This sense of confidence and pride in my appearance had a profound effect on every aspect of my world. I began to realize that in the past, the only thing

12

truly preventing me from being happy and fulfilling every aspect of my dream was merely my conception of myself. Once I realized that I didn't need to keep buying into the unhealthy and consuming expectation of appearance, my own job performance started to thrive.

Much to my surprise, my new hairstyle was also beginning to have a major influence on others in my life. After witnessing my transformation physically, professionally and personally, many of my closest friends and colleagues made the decision to give up their relaxers too and go natural. It was also an amazing feeling to be the only natural woman in the room at times. Men often walked up to me and said *"I love your hair"*, *"Damn, you're looking fine,* or *"Can I touch your puff?"* Finally, I had come to terms with my kinky tresses.

Of course, it was all nonsense. I never needed a wig in the first place to be accepted at my job or to be considered attractive. I just had to be myself and learn to accept my own, natural hair for what it was – a beautiful and real part and reflection of who I am as a person and as a black woman. *13*

Although my transition was fraught with many difficult moments, I grew tremendously from this experience. Today, I don't think twice about wearing my hair natural and have finally come to fully appreciate the beauty and uniqueness of my kinky mane. When I put on my favorite suit and walk into a client meeting, I know it doesn't matter how I wear my hair. My opinions will be respected and heard. My relationships with my colleagues, both black and white, have never been better. And, strangely enough, some of our most interesting conversations have been about the uniqueness and beauty of black hair.

My natural journey has taught me many lessons -- but most importantly, that we, as black woman, must embrace our unique differences and traits and no longer be ashamed of who we truly are. It has taken me close to twenty-five years to accept my hair for what it really is, but now, I can now finally say, THANK GOD I'M NATURAL!

Check out my Michael Jackson baby hair and my freshly permed locks. Wow, I was definitely doing it back in the 1st grade.

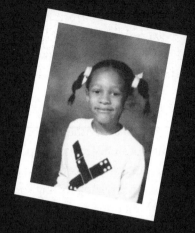

14

Remember the french roll? This 90s throwback was a black girl favorite for every high school dance.

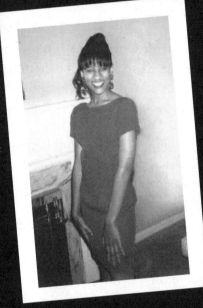

I owe Halle big time for making this short sexy do popular and providing me with temporary relief from my life long obsession with long flowing tresses.

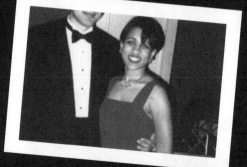

Here I am kickin' it with one of my bestfriends from law school just before I did the Big Chop. I know the chin length bob looks kind of fly, but it was burning a major hole in my wallet.

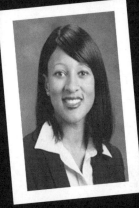

Can you even tell I am wearing a wig in this picture? Probably not. This photograph is from when I worked at my first law firm and was trying to get my Claire Huxtable on.

THANK GOD I'M NATURAL!!!

Chapter 2

Myths & Misconceptions

So, you're thinking about going natural, but you're scared that you're not mixed with enough white, Indian, or Creole to make this work? Well, not too long ago, I was worried about the very same thing. Growing up, I always thought (incorrectly) that natural hair was reserved for the Alicia Keys types. Fortunately, I came across the website www.nappturality.com, which dispelled the myth that women born with tightly coiled hair have no alternative to relaxers. Unfortunately, this myth is still widespread within our community due to lack of information about caring for our kinky tresses.

In order to help you get a handle on such misconceptions, I've tried to anticipate most, if not all, of your concerns in the following section. My hope is that this reality check will help to eliminate some of your worries and give you the confidence to get started on your own natural journey.

Myth #1 - Natural Hair is only for those with Good Hair

This old school belief has been passed down from generation to generation. But believe me, times have changed. Turn on the TV and you can't go ten minutes without seeing a black woman with a twist out or a freeform fro in a national television commercial. Flip through the pages of Cosmo, Vogue, and Essence and you'll also see black women with all different skin tones and hair textures rocking the latest fashions! It doesn't matter if your curls are loose and wavy or tight and kinky. *Natural hair is the look of the day and can be worn by just about anyone.*

Myth #2 - Natural Hair is Unmanageable

Nothing could be further from the truth. The media and relaxer manufacturers have done an excellent job of tricking us all into believing that our natural hair requires a miracle simply to maintain. Check out the ads in this month's *Ebony* and I promise that you'll find pages of relaxer advertisements that promise longer, silkier, and easier to manage hair. It should come as no surprise that these corporations have profited to the tune of billions of dollars by perpetuating such myths and preying on the insecurities of black women everywhere. The truth is that natural hair is just as manageable as relaxed hair and often gives the wearer greater freedom and flexibility. Once you've mastered the basic grooming techniques and have found products that your hair likes/responds to, caring for your natural tresses will be as easy as A, B, C.

Myth #3 - Natural Hair is Dirty

Most naturals are apt to wash their hair more frequently, not less -- because many natural styles can be easily redone at home. For most women with relaxed hair, this is clearly not an option. The fear of ruining their wrap or roller set often prevents them from enjoying this basic, but essential luxury. So, if you really want to let go of all your hair worries, skip the relaxers and go natural. You can enjoy long hot showers, walks in the rain or whatever you wish -- and still wear your hair just the way you like.

For Chynna, of Atlanta, Georgia, "The best part about being natural is having the freedom to jump in the shower after working out and wash your hair without any worries." It's like having your cake and eating it too. *For those of you who don't know, a "natural" is someone who has decided to wear their hair in its natural state – without a chemical relaxer, texturizers or other texture altering treatments. As you continue reading, flip to the glossary in the back of the book if you come across other terms with which you're unfamiliar.*

Myth #4 - Natural Hair is Dry and Hard

"When I first went natural, my hair looked and felt like Brillo!" stated Kameron from Washington D.C. But like so many other women, Kameron found that with time (and healing) her hair texture changed. As you start to transition, your hair may indeed feel dry and brittle. After years of perming, your hair and hair follicles need the chance to recover from all the damage caused by those harsh chemicals. Trust me, once your follicles have healed, your hair will began to feel soft and supple again. *Another tip:* using products specially formulated for curly or color treated hair will help to keep your hair conditioned and well moisturized.

Myth #5 - Natural Hair is only for the Political/Spiritual Types

I love me some Angela Davis -- but natural hair is for everyone. Although the Afro was once a symbol for political change, today, being natural is nothing more than a hairstyle. Natural hair looks just as good on women wearing their dashikis and head wraps as it does on women sporting their St. John suits. At the end of the day, you're an individual and natural hair can't take that away from you.

Myth #6 - Natural Hair is Unprofessional

I've heard this a thousand times before. Sadly enough, we as black women are more likely than our white counterparts to view our kinky tresses as unprofessional or inferior. I personally have not experienced any problems with being natural and working for one of the top law firms in the country. In fact, I have found it much easier to be myself around my colleagues and clients sporting natural hair rather than with perms and wigs. *Go figure!!*

A word of caution: different fields have different standards when it comes to determining what constitutes "professional". In some professions, like advertising and retail, black women have greater freedom to be creative with their style of dress and hair. "My co-workers love my fro-hawk," Felicia, a columnist at a top fashion magazine, confided. But such styles are far more daring and may not fit with your employer's culture if you work at a bank, law firm, doctor's office, etc. Just remember to use your best judgment and as always, feel free to contact me if you have any questions or need advice.

19

Myth #7 - Your Styling Options are Limited

Once upon a time, tight, braided styles were our only options when it came to wearing our hair natural. But times have changed. Now, there are so many looks to choose from. Not only do you have the option to wear your hair straight or curly -- but you can also experiment with cornrows, flat twists, Bantu knots, comb coils, roller sets, and twist outs. If you're feeling modern and funky, you can rock a blow out or pay homage to Pam Grier, the original Foxy Cleopatra, and sport a big-ass Afro. For a look that is timeless and sophisticated, you can never go wrong with slicking your hair back into a bun. And, of course, I can't forget to give a shout-out to all the ladies with the Teeny Weeny Afros. Color is also a great way to spice up your look and give yourself more variety. Remember, variety is the spice of life and with natural hair, you're never short on seasoning.

Myth #8 - You Can Have a Texturizer and Still be Natural

To be quite clear: "natural hair" is hair that hasn't been chemically straightened. Your hair isn't natural if you use a texturizer or a chemical relaxer. These products alter the chemical makeup of your hair and straighten and/or loosen your natural curls. The same is true for no-lye relaxers and hair softeners. Some naturals, however, choose to wear their hair straight, using a heated styling appliance instead of relaxers. In my opinion, these women are still by definition considered natural.

Myth #9 – You'll Never Get a Date with Natural Hair

This is so untrue! Most brothas I know are definitely feeling the natural hair thing. Many naturals find that men are drawn to them because their hair is so different and unique. Renee from Baltimore explains, "When I was sporting the long, black weave, I definitely got a different kind of attention. Now, I'm some kind of beautiful black queen, even though the only thing that changed was my hair."

Myth #10 - Natural Hair Doesn't Need to be Trimmed

This couldn't be further from the truth. Although natural hair is less prone to breakage and split ends, it should be trimmed every six to eight weeks. Regular trims will also keep your mane healthy and looking its best.

Myth #11 - Natural Hair is Stronger than Relaxed Hair

Although natural hair can typically withstand greater stress and abuse, this doesn't mean you can flat iron your hair straight everyday or comb your hair when it's dry with a rat-tail comb. Your natural hair will break off! Remember, kinky hair is delicate and should always be handled gently and with care.

Myth #12 - Black Hair Doesn't Grow Long

All hair -- white and black -- grows about one-half inch per month. "If your hair does not get longer, it is not because it is not growing, but because it continually breaks," says Harvard trained dermatologist Dr. Susan Taylor and author of the best selling book *Brown Skin.*

Unfortunately, black women continue to fight a never-ending battle with breakage and over-processed hair caused by chemical relaxers and harsh styling practices (e.g. weaves, tight braids, etc.). Many women find, however, that going natural helps to minimize breakage. Some naturals even report that their hair is healthier and grows longer and thicker than ever before.

Myth #13 - Petroleum and Lanolin are Good for the Hair

Here's my rule of thumb: if it looks like you can fry chicken in it or petroleum and/or lanolin are listed among the first five ingredients on the label, don't buy it. Petroleum and lanolin based products clog your pores and leave your hair feeling greasy and coated. Instead, look for products that are light in texture and contain natural oils, like jojoba, sesame and sunflower oils. These ingredients are easily absorbed by your strands and keep the hair soft and shiny.

Myth #14 - Water is Bad for Your Hair

The truth is that natural hair craves moisture -- because the natural *21* oils produced by the scalp have a hard time traveling down the spiral hair strand. Misting your hair with water every two to three days will keep your natural hair feeling soft and supple.

Myth #15 - Natural Hair Requires No Maintenance

"There is no such thing as no-maintenance black hair," says Symone Hilton, owner of Natural Trendsetters Salon in Ft. Lauderdale, Florida. It doesn't matter if you are rocking a TWA or sporting locks, you'll still need to keep your hair and scalp clean and well conditioned -- and your ends trimmed to achieve a healthy mane.

Key Points To Remember

- Natural hair can be worn by those with even the kinkiest hair types.
- Natural hair *is* professional.
- Natural hair *is* versatile.
- Caring for natural hair is easy, with the right products and styling tools.

22

23

Chapter 3
A Brush With History

A hairstyle is just a hairstyle, right? Wrong! Choices we make about our hair, clothes and the way we tend to our bodies are connected to our deeply embedded, yet mostly invisible, perceptions about ourselves, our identity, and our place in society at large. When a majority of young black women believe that they must wear their hair straight in order to succeed socially and professionally, there's clearly a problem. Fortunately, we can understand how these beliefs have evolved and come to have so much power over us. Then, we can choose to abandon them and celebrate the beauty and power that is truly our birthright. So, take a little stroll with me through history to find out how these negative perceptions of black hair came to be -- and how issues of race and beauty have impacted our personal choices for generations.

Slavery in America

Before Dark & Lovely, the pressing comb, or the North Atlantic slave trade, Africans celebrated the richness and beauty of their natural hair. Using mud, clay and butters and decorative combs, beads and shells, black women took great pride in creating impressive styles -- which many would classify as high art.[1] In pre-slavery Africa, a woman's hairstyle marked important life events, such as puberty, marriage or the birth of a new child. Her hair was also inevitably tied to her identity and reflected her age, social status, religion and tribal affiliation.

25

Indeed, throughout Africa, hair took on many different meanings. In Ethiopia, women, let their hair grow long as a symbol of beauty and well-being. Among the Yoruba of Nigeria, however, it was common practice for a female's head to be shaved shortly after birth to mark her emergence from the spiritual realm and again at death to signify her return.[2] In West Africa and other parts of the continent, complex braided hairstyles were typically worn by female royalty and other high-ranking officials to signify power and status in ancient communities. Sadly, many of these magnificent grooming practices didn't survive the horror and brutality of slavery.

When the Africans arrived in America, they lacked both the time and implements to create such elaborate hairstyles. Slaveholders gave very little consideration to the personal hygiene needs of their property and generally viewed time spent on grooming as an unnecessary distraction from the work at hand. For some slaves, the carving of a comb resulted in punishment. In some extreme cases, the consequences was death.[3]

Under these conditions, the Africans' hair often went unkempt and scalp diseases, such as lice and ringworm, flourished among slave populations. Whereas in Africa, women spent hours every day grooming and styling their hair, in America black women frequently covered their hair out of shame and embarrassment. Over time, however, slave owners gradually recognized the health and economic benefits associated with good hygiene. As a result, some slaves were given regular opportunities to care for their hair.

Work assignments also significantly influenced the amount of time slaves spent on grooming. Women who toiled long days in the fields had very little free time to style their tresses and usually wore scarves and head rags to prevent their locks from drying out under the scorching sun. On the other hand, slaves who worked in the master's house as laundresses, cooks, and nursemaids were required to appear neat and well groomed. These slaves had frequent contact with their owners and typically wore their hair in tight braids, plaits, or cornrows. Slave owners frequently gave preference to lighter skinned blacks with European features in assigning them the highly coveted, indoor positions -- while leaving the more strenuous outdoor jobs to darker skinned blacks.[4] Since the distinction between house slaves and field slaves was based largely on physical appearance, this sense of favoritism contributed greatly to the perception that opportunity and privilege were connected to European beauty.

By the time slavery ended, many blacks were willing to go to great lengths to emulate and achieve the same styles worn by their white owners. Using readily available household products, black women became extremely adept at developing new ways to straighten their naturally curly hair. In *Hair Story*, Ayana Byrd describes how black women "would slather the[ir] hair with butter, bacon fat, or goose grease and then use a butter knife heated in a can over a crude fire as a curling iron."[5] Axle grease intended for wagon wheels was another tool, which functioned both as a hair straightener and a hair dye. Slave mothers also developed a technique known as "banding" -- where their daughters' hair was combed free of tangles and wrapped with strips of fabric to stretch out their natural curls. As these methods improved, hair straightening became a more routine aspect in black women's lives.

Reconstruction

Skin color and hair type continued to be divisive issues in the black community long after slavery ended. During this period of economic prosperity, many blacks were desperate to change their hair texture or skin color, believing such transformations would result in economic opportunities and social advantage.[6] This insidious form of color discrimination often prevented darker skinned blacks from obtaining high-paying jobs, attending quality schools, and joining the social circles occupied by the mulatto or light skinned elite. The adherence to and acceptance of white, slave owner values fostered an environment in which the importance of hair straightening was stressed and set the stage for centuries of internal colorism and strained relationships between light and dark skinned blacks.

27

The black woman's growing obsession with *"good"* hair and light skin also made her an easy target for manufacturers of hair straighteners and skin bleaching creams in the years that followed. White companies profited handsomely from advertisements in Negro newspapers, which implied that black women could achieve class mobility and social acceptance by changing their physical appearance.[7] At the turn of the century, the pages of most Colored newspapers were filled with advertisements for skin bleaching creams and hair straighteners that read: *"You too can look lighter, brighter, and be more popular." "Get the lighter, brighter skin you've always wanted." "Turn your short, kinky, harsh and ugly hair into long, straight, beautiful hair that everyone admires." "Long, Beautiful Hair Made all the Difference."*

Many black activists, such as Booker T. Washington and Marcus Garvey, decried hair straightening and skin bleaching for their increasingly debilitating effect on the psyche and self-esteem of the Negro race. The black church was another source of strong opposition to these practices. They asserted that if God meant for blacks to have straight hair, He would have endowed them with it.[8] Yet, this was a view not shared by the majority of black women. By this time, straightened hair had become a practical necessity for women of color – who sought to prosper in mainstream, white society.

1920s – 1950s

The turn of the century brought a proliferation of hair products and styling aids, such as: Curl-I-Cure, KKK, and Ploughs -- which promised to improve the texture and manageability of black hair. The rapid growth in the black hair care industry also created opportunities for black entrepreneurs, such as the late Madame C.J. Walker (1867-1919), who is best known as the first black female millionaire. Like most black women who grew up in the postbellum South, Madame Walker "had been bombarded with messages that she was unattractive, that her frizzy, brittle hair was ugly and unsightly, [and] that her skin color rendered powerless."[9]

Although Walker popularized the use of the pressing comb, she adopted a different approach from that of her white counterparts to sell and market her products. Instead of telling black women that they needed to straighten their hair to be considered attractive, Walker crafted a message that communicated the importance of giving one's hair proper attention and taking pride in a woman's unique personal appearance. Despite the black community's continued emphasis on conforming to European beauty standards, black women were finally receiving a positive message about their own self-care and image.

By the mid-1920s, black women were using the pressing comb to straighten their hair on a regular basis. Within black communities, straightened hair became a symbol of upward mobility, which further distanced blacks from the institutions of slavery. As one woman explained, "Straightened was respectable. It was what we did . . . decent people. We don't look unkempt."[10] Black mothers also taught their daughters the importance of hair straightening at a very early age. Having grown up in the 1950s, Juadine Henderson recalls the emphasis on having straight hair throughout her childhood:

You always knew that it was not a good thing to have nappy hair. You always straightened it. One of the first things you learned about

*taking care of your own hair was how to straighten it. . . I always
knew once you washed your hair, until it was straightened, you put
a scarf on it.* [11]

Black is Beautiful

Between the 1960s and 1970s, a large majority of black women
abandoned the press and curl and other conventional beauty practices
in favor of more natural styles like the Afro. In its early beginnings, the
Afro was most commonly embraced by your typical soul sistah seen
sporting her dashiki at civil rights meetings and protest demonstrations.
Eventually, the style would gain mainstream acceptance and would be
worn simply as a fashion statement. As one magazine from the era puts
it, "Suddenly it had become fashionable to be black."[12]

The Afro, however, was not without its critics. When Stephanie
Cunningham left home to attend college at Boston University with her
close-cropped natural, her mother admonished, "You're not going to let
those white people see your hair like that!" Many black parents feared
the Afro would jeopardize their child's chances for advancement or, even
worse, cause them to be labeled as "militant" or "anti-establishment".
Many whites also viewed the style as a form of rebellion and a rejection
of Anglo Saxon standards of beauty -- which for most African-Americans
were nearly impossible to attain. Although the "Black is Beautiful"
movement was short-lived, this period offered African-Americans the
opportunity to embrace the uniqueness of their natural hair and celebrate
their heritage-- which they had long sought to (or been forced to) deny.

The Present

When corporate America opened its doors to blacks in the late
1970's and early 1980's, many blacks adopted conservative hairstyles to
increase their chances for professional advancement. Despite our progress
since then, one of the nation's historically black colleges (HBCU) made
headlines recently when they banned business majors from wearing
cornrows and locks. "When we look at the top 75 African-Americans in
corporate America, we don't see any of them with extreme hairdos,"[13] says
one university official, who believed the new policy was necessary to help
students succeed in a corporate environment.

The university's decision was met with a firestorm of criticism -- but also garnered the support of many individuals who felt "self-expression" simply did not belong in the workplace. In spite of its long-standing history of academic excellence, the policy of this HBCU reinforces the belief that we must emulate a white beauty aesthetic in order to be accepted by white America. This principle has been passed down from generation to generation since slavery and has continued to impact the way in which African-Americans perceive their own natural beauty, even today.

Black women are among the most beautiful women in the world, yet society has sought to conceal this obvious fact for centuries.[14] As women of color, we have been tricked into believing that our hair in its natural state is unmanageable, unprofessional and – even worse -- unattractive. This racist pathology is ingrained into our culture and can be traced back to the institution of slavery. Although names like Curl-I-Cure, KKK and Plough's have long been replaced by brands such as Dark & Lovely, Affirm, and Motions, the underlying message sadly remains the same – black hair is unmanageable and aesthetically inferior in its kinky state. This point is quite significant.

As we continue to learn about ourselves, we can better appreciate the impact that historical events have had on our perceptions of identity, especially as it relates to hair. Once we accept our natural texture for what it is, we can more fully embrace the true beauty that lies within. As you turn the page and embark on this journey of self-acceptance, please know that there is no greater feeling than being able to celebrate the beauty that represents the natural you!

The Greatest Moments In Kinky Hair History

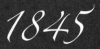 **1845**
Welcome the invention of the hot comb in, where else, France!

 1910
Madam C.J. Walker, the first self-made, black female millionaire, makes her first appearance in the Guinness Book of World Records.

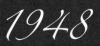 **1948**
The Mexican chemist, Jose Calva, discovers the first "relaxer." The same chemical process that makes sheep's wool super soft also makes kinky hair straight.

 1969
A picture of Angela Davis wearing a huge Afro ——is disseminated to the masses by the FBI. The message: black women with Afros are dangerous.

 1971
Hair and politics makes the news. Melba Tolliver is fired from an ABC affiliate. Why? She wore an Afro while covering Tricia Nixon's wedding. Shocking!

 1981
The American Health and Beauty Aids Institute introduces the proud lady symbol, reminding consumers to buy black.

 1984
While filming a commercial for Pepsi-Cola, the King of Pop Michael Jackson's hair catches fire.

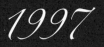 **1989**
Quaker Oats gives Aunt Jemima a makeover. They get rid of her familiar red head-rag and replace it with a fresh (and toxic) no-lye relaxer do.

1997
On her debut album, "Baduism," Singer Erykah Badu rocks the world by posing on the cover with her head wrapped, ushering in a new era of Afro-centric styles.

1998

Brooklyn, NY, a white teacher is threatened with bodily harm as a result of reading a book titled, "Nappy Hair," to her third-grade students. She finally leaves the school out of fear for her safety. The book then goes on to sell a hundred thousand copies.

1999

People Magazine names Grammy award-winning singer Lauryn Hill one of its "50 Most Beautiful People." What made it news to us? Her tresses were locked.

When some of her signature beads fly off the ends of her braids and land on the court at the Australian Open, tennis-star, Venus Williams, receives a point penalty.

2007

CBS gives veteran radio talk show host Don Imus the boot after he refers to the Rutgers University Women's Basketball team as "nappy-headed ho's," while on the air. His comments leads to high-profile public protests and many of his major sponsors abandoning him and his show.

Key Points to Remember

- We can overcome our struggles with hair and identity by learning from our past.

- Africans celebrated the richness and beauty of natural hair before arriving in America.

- Black women's identity/sense of beauty was greatly impacted by the institution of slavery.

- Hair straightening has been passed down from generation to generation due to a fundamental lack of knowledge and information.

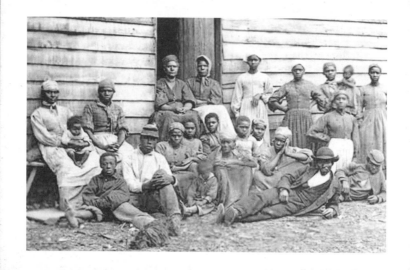

Slavery

As seen in this photo taken in 1862, female slaves kept their hair constantly covered, in part, to protect it from the scorching heat, but also out of shame and embarrassment due to their natural texture.

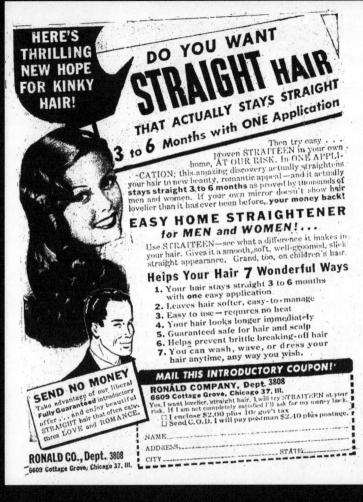

1930s

As black women, we've all given up on our tresses at times, but this ad reminds us that all hope is not lost for those of us born with kinky hair.

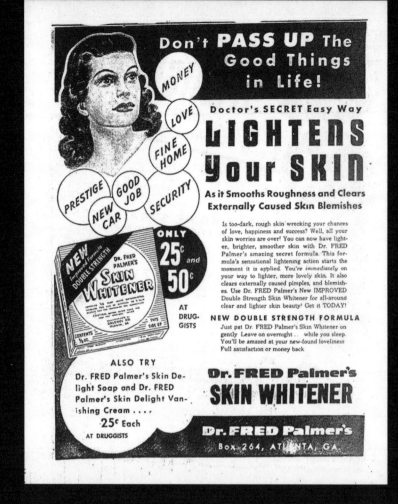

36

1940s

It doesn't get any more obvious then this. This advertisement from the early 1940s makes clear that everything in life that matters -- money, love, a good job, security and a home – depend on your complexion.

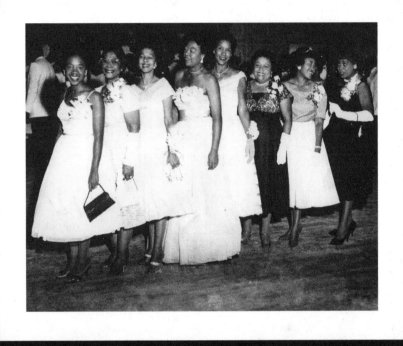

1950s

By the mid 1950s, straight hair was prized over kinky textures so much so that a large majority of black women adopted the press and curl as the style of choice as seen in this photograph.

Chapter 4

Anatomy 101

Knowledge of the elemental details about your kinky tresses is essential to choosing the right styling products and protecting your hair from long-term damage and abuse. So, let's get down to business! **Welcome to Hair 101.**

Hair is composed almost entirely of protein and is the fastest growing tissue in the human body, second only to bone marrow. Our hair's primary function is protection. It protects the scalp from sunburn and injury and also helps to regulate body temperature.

Hair grows at the rate of one-half inch per month, on average. Obviously, this isn't a universal law since growth rates vary from person to person and are affected by diet, stress and other factors. However, many black women complain that their hair never grows. The truth is that kinky hair is extremely delicate and prone to breakage. So in reality, your strands may be growing and then snapping right off. The use of chemical relaxers, even the ones that claim to be gentle, can also leave the hair weak and more prone to breakage.

39

Remember that box of relaxer sitting, oh so innocently, on the drug store shelf? Right next to it is the box of *Heal Your Hair*. Coincidence? I think not. This is why we must learn to handle our natural hair gently and with utmost care.

* * * *

All hair is comprised of two basic parts: the follicle and the shaft. This is true for any person – regardless of his or her race.

Hair Follicle

The hair follicle is a tiny sac that lies below the surface of the skin from which the hair shaft grows. Each hair follicle contains three to five sebaceous glands that secrete a natural conditioner (sebum), which keeps the hair soft and moisturized. Generally speaking, black women have curved hair follicles, which is why our hair is typically curly instead of straight. Black hair also tends to be dry and require extra moisture and conditioning since the oil produced by the scalp doesn't travel down the curved follicle or curled strand as freely as it does in

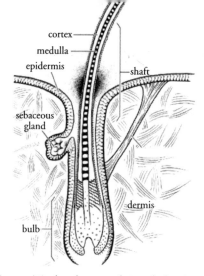

Hair Follicle

straight hair. Dr. Susan Taylor has explained that since black women's hair is usually drier, they don't need to wash their hair as frequently as white women do.

At the base of each hair follicle is the *dermal papilla*. The dermal papilla provides the follicle with nourishment from the bloodstream and plays an important role in the hair's growth and development. So long as the dermal papilla is healthy and well nourished, it will continue to produce stunningly beautiful hair at a fairly even growth rate.

Hair Shaft

The hair shaft is fully visible above the scalp and is comprised of three parts: the cuticle, the cortex, and the medulla. The cuticle forms the outermost layer of the hair shaft and is made up of thin overlapping cells, which resemble fish scales. Heat styling and harsh chemicals, like relaxers and color, will adversely affect the growth and natural development of the cuticle. If the cuticle is in good condition, the hair will feel smooth and give off a healthy shine. If the cuticle is badly damaged, the hair will feel coarse and brittle -- and may tangle easily. For this reason, most hair products are designed to treat this layer.

Cortex

The cortex is composed of rope-like fibers and forms the middle layer of the hair shaft. The strength, elasticity, texture, and color of the hair are all determined by the composition of this layer. Relaxers, texturizers, hair dyes and heat straightening all work by altering the chemical bonds found in the cortex. In the case of relaxers and hair color, the change to the cortex is permanent. This is not the case with blow drying and flat ironing, which straighten the hair temporarily through heat application rather than a chemical one.

Medulla

Lastly, the medulla is the innermost layer, which is composed almost entirely of soft protein. The medulla plays a very insignificant role in the hair's growth and development. This layer isn't effected by products or styling processes and is even known to be absent in some hair strands. Phew! Isn't it a relief to know there is at least one part of your hair is immune to all of this trouble?

So by now, you should understand how the basic structure of your hair will affect the choices you make from here on out -- in terms of how you'll care for your hair in the future. It's my hope that by being armed with this information, you'll be able to make better, more *41* informed decisions about how to best care for you own mane. As a result, not only will your tresses look healthier but they will actually *be* healthier.

Hair Facts

- There are approximately 100,000 hairs on your head.

- We lose on average between 50-100 hairs per day due to normal shedding.

- Each follicle will produce about 20 hairs in your lifetime.

- During pregnancy, your hair grows longer and thicker because of the high estrogen levels in your blood.

- As you age, some of your follicles lose their ability to produce hair.

- Hair is comprised almost 25% of water. The moisture content is responsible for the suppleness and elasticity of your strands.

Chapter 5

Type & Texture

At first glance, all the hair on your head looks the same, right? However, when you take a closer look in the mirror, you'll see that your strands can range from kinky to straight and everything in between. When we use words like "kinky", "curly", "wavy" and "straight", we're referring to hair type. Hair type is determined by the curvature of your hair follicles (remember them?), which come in all shapes and sizes. So many of us fall into the dangerous mindset of wanting a hair type different than our own. Knowing your own hair type, however, will help you to better care for your tresses and maximize your styling options. Most importantly, embracing the hair type you were born with and learning to care for it with love will bring you one step closer to having the glorious natural crown you always dreamed of.

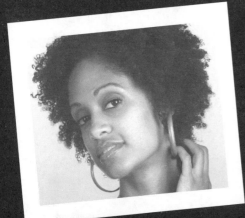

Kinky Hair

Like most black women, I have what many people consider to be kinky hair. Kinky hair is related to curly hair in that it is tightly coiled. Kinky hair can have a clearly visible curl pattern, which ranges from pencil size curls to coffee-stirrer s-shaped coils. Because it is tightly coiled, kinky hair can shrink up to 80% of its actual length.

43

Although this hair type appears to be thick and strong, it is actually quite delicate and highly susceptible to breakage. Of all the hair types, kinky hair has the fewest cuticle layers, which means it has the least amount of protection. Kinky hair doesn't usually have much of a shine. But with proper care, you can achieve a healthy sheen. One of the best things about this hair type is that it actually has great hold. This allows it to be styled and manipulated in many different ways – with great results.

Curly Hair

Curly hair comes in all shapes and sizes -- from large bouncy Shirley Temple ringlets to small tight coils about the size of a pencil or a straw. Curly hair doesn't have much of a shine because the hair's surface isn't smooth and doesn't reflect a great deal of light. It is also prone to dryness since it's difficult for the natural oils produced by the scalp to travel down the curled hair shaft. Humidity will also make this hair type curlier. Curly hair, however, isn't prone to shrink as much as kinky hair. This hair type has tons of body and is truly great for experimenting with different styles.

44

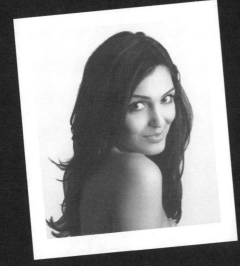

Wavy Hair

Wavy hair has a long S-shaped pattern, which falls somewhere between curly hair and straight hair. This hair type stays well moisturized and usually lies flat against the head. Wavy hair reflects light well, so it usually has more of a natural shine than kinky or curly hair.

45

Straight Hair

Straight hair doesn't have a wave or curl pattern. This hair type also tends to be oily and must be shampooed frequently to prevent it from attracting dirt and looking limp. While naturally straight hair is the least prone to breakage, it can also be the most difficult to work with since it doesn't hold styles well.

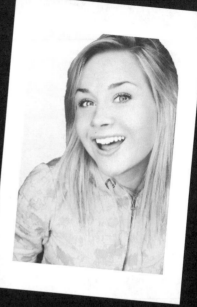

46

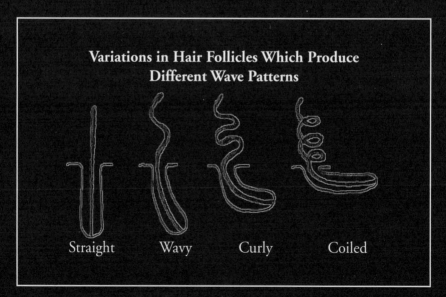

Variations in Hair Follicles Which Produce Different Wave Patterns

Straight   Wavy   Curly   Coiled

Finding Your Texture

Now that you have a handle on your hair type, you'll need to learn about your hair's texture. Hair comes in a variety of textures. Hair that shines gives off a sharp reflection of light, while hair that has sheen gives off a dull reflection. Generally speaking, shine is a common characteristic of straight hair and sheen is an attribute of curly hair. It can make things simpler to make up categories, with lists of different hair characteristics:

Thready Hair is generally not all that shiny but will appear very shiny if you pull it tight into a braid or a bun. Thready hair is low frizz. It's easy to get wet and quick drying, too.

Wiry Hair sparkles erratically because of the shape of each strand. It's thought to have relatively low shine and frizz. You can never fully wet this kind of hair all the way through, because water only beads up and rolls off the hair strands.

Cottony Hair is super high frizz, like a ball of cotton! It has a low sheen on its own but, if the hair is pulled tight, it will appear to have a high shine. This kind of hair will absorb water quickly -- but if you want to get it thoroughly wet you have to really soak it, squeezing the water into the hair. *47*

Spongy Hair has high sheen but low shine and compact frizz. It absorbs water before it gets thoroughly wet.

Silky Hair has very high shine and can range from having lots of frizz to having none. It wets easily in water.

Feeling confused? Well don't worry! There are lots of folks out there currently coming up with great ways to make all of this a lot simpler for you.

Classification Systems (Andre Walker and LOIS)

Several efforts have been made recently to classify the variety of black hair types/textures -- using different naming and numbering systems.

Unfortunately, no one system fully captures the diversity of hair textures and types that exist among this racial group. Some naturals, however, find it useful to know what category their hair falls into when discussing product recommendations and their personal experiences with their hair online.

Oprah Winfrey's personal stylist, Andre Walker, has developed a numbering system to classify different hair types, which is frequently used among naturals to converse about their tresses. In his book, *Andre Talks Hair*, Walker assigns a number 1-4 to different hair types. These hair types include straight, wavy, curly and kinky. On this scale, the number 1 refers to hair that is completely straight and has no curl pattern and the number 4 describes hair which is tightly coiled and fairly common among black women. Walker then assigns a letter to each number to denote how curly the hair is, with 'A' being the straightest, 'B' having more of a curl, and so on.

48 Many naturals believe that Walker's system doesn't address the fact that women with kinky or curly hair can also have a combination of different hair types and textures on their head. Some naturals have suggested that there may be a need for additional subcategories for the curly and kinky hair types. Despite its limitations, Walker's method is currently considered the first of its kind -- and one of the best available hair classification systems to date.

The founder of www.Ourhair.net has also developed another extremely helpful hair typing system called LOIS. The LOIS system is wonderful because it focuses specifically on black hair.

When it comes to taking care of your natural hair, it is important to understand what you are working with. This basic knowledge can help you choose products and styles that will keep your hair looking its best. Although there is no single product that will satisfy the hair care needs of all black women, understanding the special characteristics of black hair will help you to better care for your tresses. Finally, there is no such thing as "*good hair*" or "*bad hair*". At the end of the day, what matters the most is that your hair is healthy and in great condition.

The Andre Walker System

Andre Walker, world renowned hair expert and Oprah Winfrey's personal stylist, has developed a hair classification system based on hair type that is frequently referenced online in chatrooms and message boards related to natural hair care.

Type 1: Straight Hair. Type 1 hair is straight with no curl or wave pattern and is more common among Caucasians and Asians than those of African descent. This hair type can be extremely resistant to curling and shaping and has a tendency to be shiny and oily.

Type 2: Wavy Hair. Walker classifies hair that has a noticeable wave pattern, but little or no curl as Type 2 hair. This hair type tends to lie flat against the scalp and will have long S shaped curves. Type 2 hair has very little body but can be given an instant lift with the right haircut and combination of styling products. There are three Type 2 subtypes: A, fine and thin; B, medium-textured; and C, thick and coarse. Notable Type 2's: Mariah Carey and Chili from TLC.

Type 3: Curly Hair. Type 3 hair has a well-defined S-pattern and is the hair type in which the hair begins to be classified as curly. Curly hair is not as shiny as straight or wavy hair -- but it does have a lot more body. It is not uncommon for type 3's to have multiple textures on their head with the crown being the curliest. Walker classifies those with large shiny curls as Type 3As, while 3Bs have curls that range in size from ringlets to corkscrews. Type 3C hair has smaller curls and may appear to be slightly kinky. Famous Type 3s: Alicia Keys, Kelis and Tracey Ellis Ross.

Type 4: Kinky Hair. Walker classifies hair that is kinky and tightly curled as Type 4 hair. At first glance, kinky hair appears to be coarse. In reality, it is extremely fine -- with many strands densely packed together. Kinky hair is also drier and has less of a shine than other hair types. Walker also divides kinky hair into subcategories based on curl pattern. Type 4A hair has a clearly defined "S" shaped curl pattern, which ranges from pen size curls to coffee-stirrer size S-shaped coils. Type 4B hair has the same characteristics as Type 4A hair, but has a tighter wave pattern and kinks of various size. Instead of an S-shaped curl pattern, 4B hair will usually have a Z-shape. Notable type 4's: Angela Bassett, Oprah Winfrey, Macy Gray, Lauryn Hill, Floetry, India Arie and Jill Scott.

For more information about Walker's classification system, check out his book, *Andre Talks Hair.*

The LOIS System

How to determine which daughter (or son) of LOIS you are:

Remove a single strand of the most common type of hair on your head. If you have different textures (most of us do), use a strand that reflects the most common texture on your head.

The hair should be freshly washed -- without products applied to it and rinsed in cold water. Or, gently rinse a single hair with a little dish detergent and rinse in cold water.

Lay the hair on an absorbent paper towel to dry. When the hair is completely dry, look at the pattern without touching it.

- If the hair has all bends, right angles and folds with little to no curve, then you are daughter L.

- If the strand is rolled up into the shape of one or several zeros like a spiral, then you are daughter O.

- If the hair lies mostly flat with no distinctive curve or bend, you are daughter I.

- If the strand looks like a wavy line with hills and valleys, then you are daughter S.

It will be common to have a combination of the LOIS letters, (with more dominant) which can help you determine which daughter of LOIS you are. If you cannot see one letter over the others, then combine the letters.

Key Points to Remember

- Black hair textures and types can vary widely, even on a single head.

- There are four basic hair types -- straight, wavy, curly, and kinky.

- Knowing your hair type will allow you to choose products and styles that keep your tresses looking and feeling their best.

51

Chapter 6

Relaxers
How Safe Are They?

Before I took the plunge and went natural, I could never imagine myself with a chunky fro or two strand twists. But now, I feel my kinky tresses fit my outgoing personality. Despite the numerous advantages of going natural, many black women still can't fathom the possibility of giving up their relaxers. This is due largely to the fact that most of us don't know the first thing about caring for our natural hair. We've been so brainwashed into believing that our natural texture is socially unacceptable that we often choose to endure a lifetime of scalp burns, hair loss and never ending breakage all in the name of beauty (not to mention the extreme financial burden).

The truth is, we have options -- lots of them. You don't need a relaxer to wear your hair straight or a texturizer to enhance your natural curl pattern. All you need is patience and a basic understanding of your hair type. To make it easy, I've researched how relaxers work, discovered the long-term effect these chemicals have on your body, and found the proper way to handle and care for your natural hair -- however you choose to wear it. Armed with this wealth of information, you'll hopefully be inspired to embrace your natural texture and bid farewell to relaxers for good!

How Relaxers Work

When applied to the hair, a relaxer loosens the natural curl pattern and causes the hair to soften. Some women can achieve a completely straight look with a relaxer. But for individuals with extremely curly hair, the results will be looser curls, which can then be straightened with the use of a blow dryer or curling iron. In both instances, the process is irreversible and the damage is long lasting.

In recent years, no-lye relaxers have grown in popularity. The term *"no-lye"*, however, can be very misleading. Advertising creates the impression that these products are much safer. But the fact is that all of these products have the same ill effects on the hair. Although no-lye relaxers tend to be less damaging, all relaxers contain caustic chemicals that strip away the hair's natural moisture -- leaving it dry, brittle and prone to breakage.

A common complaint among black women is that our hair never

grows. In fact, nothing could be further from the truth. Our hair doesn't achieve great lengths because it continually breaks off due to chemical treatments and improper styling habits. Using products manufactured for chemically treated hair and limiting the use of heated styling appliances can help to combat dryness and minimize breakage. Still, I ask you, why inflict the damage in the first place? If you really long for gorgeous, healthy hair, your best bet is to go natural. Giving up relaxers once and for all will make a huge difference in the health and overall condition of your hair, which you can see and feel. Plus, going natural is much easier than you think.

Are You Safe?

As consumers, we think it's safe to purchase cosmetics and beauty aids sold at our local drugstores or advertised in commercials. We believe that the FDA has our back and if for some unfortunate reason a product harms us, we'll be justly compensated (e.g. medical bills, pain and suffering, etc.). Like so many others, this is what Alicia Burton thought when she purchased the Rio Relaxer after seeing it advertised as a "gentle, all-natural chemical-free" hair straightening system.

After using Rio only three times, Burton remembers chunks of her hair coming out in handfuls. "I was devastated. In less than a week, I was completely bald." As we flipped through the pages of her high school photo album, Burton points out the pictures of the bad weave she was forced to wear to her senior prom and a photocopy of the check for (a mere) $75[15], which she received as the settlement payment in a class action suit brought against the manufacturer. Burton, who has been natural ever since, is now weary of all chemical straighteners and vows that she will never fall victim to relaxers or their "all natural" alternatives again.

Burton is just one of many women to experience the agony of hair loss as a result of using the Rio Naturalizer System. In 1994 and early 1995, the U.S. Food and Drug Administration (FDA) received more than 3,000 consumer complaints of scalp irritation, hair loss, and hair breakage from individuals who used Rio. Some women also reported that their hair turned green from trying this product. The results of an FDA investigation later showed that Rio products were more acidic than the instructions indicated. Plus, although the label described the products as *"all natural"*, they actually contained many ingredients commonly understood to be *"chemicals."*

Rio illustrates the unknown dangers all black female consumers face in their dealings with relaxer manufacturers and products, which are still widely available to the consumer. Burton, however, was lucky. Although it took nearly two years for her hair to grow back, Burton didn't suffer any permanent scalp damage. "The texture of my hair has definitely changed as a result of using Rio," she says "but I'm just fortunate to have hair at all."

Still, many women suffer far worse consequences. Isabella Broekhuizen was left permanently bald after using a relaxer, which brought her U.S. modeling career to an early end. Like Burton, the manufacturer offered to settle with Broekhuizen for $75 even though she must now wear a wig for the rest of her life and will never model again. Broekhuizen has tried to use her experience to warn other black women about the dangers of relaxers -- but many are fooled into thinking that such an unfortunate event will never happen to them.

55

Today, Broekhuizen is back at home in the Netherlands still fighting for justice. Her story is a powerful lesson about the unknown dangers of relaxers and her pictures are a constant reminder of one life that was permanently ruined by chemical straighteners. You can learn more about her case by visiting www.isab.nl or picking up a copy of her book, No Hair Left.

Many consumers, like Burton and Broekhuizen, trust that relaxer manufacturers adequately test their products for safety before they are sold to the general public. But it should come as no surprise that this is, sadly, not always the case. The FDA's position is that consumers must inform themselves of the risks associated with hair care products containing chemicals to ensure their proper use. Okay, sure -- being informed is a good idea, a smart move. But when "proper use," by a consumer has nothing to do with the fact that a product is dangerous no matter how it is used, the FDA should stand up for what is in the consumer's best interest.

Isabella Broekhuizen was on her way to becoming one of the Netherlands's top black models before using a relaxer, which left her permanently bald.

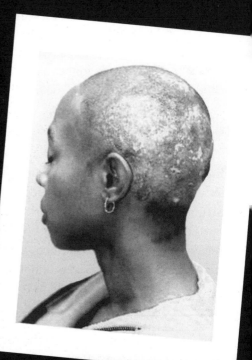

56

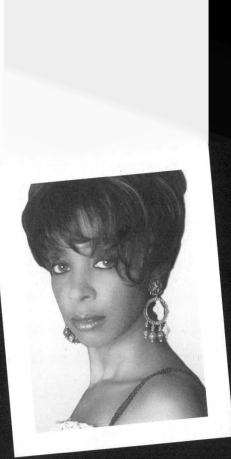

Broekhuizen must wear a wig for the rest of her life to hide the chemical burns left on her scalp after a relaxer episode gone wrong.

57

a big, fat NO! In the long run, we're much better off physically, mentally, and emotionally when we wear our hair natural, as it was intended to be. So, my advice? Go natural and count yourself lucky to be out of the fray!

The Dangers of Relaxers

I will admit, there have been significant improvements in relaxers over the years. Still, the long-term effects of applying these chemicals in close proximity to the scalp remain largely the same – **DANGEROUS AND UNKNOWN**. FDA records show that consumer complaints (relating to relaxers) range from reports of minor hair breakage to even more serious injuries -- such as scalp burns that require emergency medical attention.[16] Relaxer side effects may also include: irritation of the mucus membranes, dermatitis, coughing, thinning hair, bald spots, scalp rashes, scarring of the scalp, and permanent hair loss.[17]

While it has not yet been proven, relaxers may even increase the incidence of cancer and memory loss. What is even more alarming is that sodium hydroxide -- the active ingredient found in most relaxers -- is commonly used in everyday household products like Drano and Nair! Just think, the same harsh chemicals that are used to unclog your pipes are also considered *"safe"* by the FDA to use on your scalp!

7 Reasons to Stop Relaxing

When I sent out a mass email to my girlfriends and female business associates asking them why they went natural, I was surprised by the number of responses I received. Some of the emails had me dying laughing, while others brought me very close to tears. To give you a sense of why we are natural and lovin' it, here are seven of the most popular reasons why women are taking the plunge and giving up chemical straighteners for good.

1. Freedom

Going natural has to be the most liberating experience. The ability to live carefree without the constant worry of having the picture perfect wrap can give life a brand new meaning. "Sleeping in on Saturday mornings, working out five days a week, and not having to worry about my hair while I am on vacation were things I could never do when I was relaxed," says Kiesha from Atlanta.

Most naturals can identify with this newfound sense of freedom. As Tina from Houston puts it, "I love not having to wake up forty-five minutes earlier in the morning to make sure every strand looks perfect and is in place. Now, that I'm natural, I get up and go and my hair looks great all the time." She adds that going natural has also allowed her to spend more time with her family and work on getting her event planning business off the ground. These are just two women, who have experienced the liberating joy most of us feel once we are no longer slaves to relaxers and chemical straighteners. Taking the step may seem scary at first. But once you do, you'll wonder why you didn't make this decision sooner – trust me.

2. Hair Loss (Traction Alopecia)

Hair loss and bald spots were also issues of great concern. "I see so much hair loss at an early age now that it has become the norm," says mane pro A.J. Johnson, owner of AJES The Salon in Chicago. It's not unusual for little girls to have suffered so much hair loss caused by chemical damage that they can't even pull their hair into a ponytail. Thinning edges, breakage, and permanent hair loss are the price many black women are willing to pay for straight hair -- but it doesn't have to be this way. "Many women go natural and still wear their hair straight," continues Johnson.

3. Breakage

I've spoken with natural stylists all around the country and the general consensus is that breakage is just a normal part of using a relaxer. There is no real way around it -- but this problem has left many black women believing that our hair naturally doesn't grow long. In reality, the natural hair on our head is not one uniform texture. Some hairs are coarse and curly, while others may be loose and wavy. Using the same strength of relaxer on different textures will produce varying results. This explains why certain areas of your hair are constantly plagued by breakage despite regular care and maintenance.

4. Scalp Damage

We all know what it feels like when your relaxer starts to burn. You grit your teeth, sweat starts pouring down your face, and you just pray that you can withstand the tingling sensation long enough to get your roots straight. A few sores here and there is far better than a bad perm that will leave our hair slightly nappy, right? **WRONG**. As black women, we subject ourselves to this painful ritual every six to eight weeks for hair that is silky straight. Unfortunately, this habit has left many of us with permanent scalp damage.

5. Pregnancy

As black women become more health conscious, we have also started to consider the effect relaxers can have on our unborn children. My girlfriend Eboni told me that when she became pregnant, "My decision to stop using relaxers was a no-brainer. I wasn't going to put anything into my body that could potentially hurt my baby."

60

Although there are no studies yet that show chemical relaxers have any permanent effect on a fetus, trace amounts of these chemicals can be absorbed by the scalp into the blood stream. Dr. Shari Brasner, an obstetrician at Mount Sinai Medical Center in New York City and the author of *Advice From a Pregnant Obstetrician*, advises her patients to be "conservative in the critical first ten weeks of gestation," while some doctors discourage the use of chemial hair services for the entire duration of the pregnancy. The only way to ensure that relaxers and hair dyes do not harm the developing fetus is to discontinue their use while pregnant. *This begs the question:* Why is it so easy to make a decision for the benefit and health of our babies but not for ourselves? Don't we deserve the same level of TLC?

6. Cancer

For six decades, cigarette manufacturers denied that smoking caused cancer – a decision which made R.J. Reynolds a billionaire and cost us nearly four million lives each year.[18] Relaxers, like cigarettes, are addictive in their own way and generate billions of dollars in revenue annually. Relaxers are also like cigarettes in that it could be decades before we learn the true side effects these products have on the health and lives of black women.

Currently, there are no scientific studies that prove without a doubt an existing link between relaxers and cancer. Important insights may be drawn, however, from recent medical research that shows long term use of permanent hair dyes increases a woman's risk of bladder cancer and non-Hodgkin's lymphoma.[19] For black women who routinely use relaxers and believe these products are completely safe, this may be our only warning before it is too late.

7. Nerve Damage (Memory Loss)

With no family history of Alzheimer's Disease, 62 year old Sophie Harmon is now suffering from this terrible affliction. A long time hairdresser, her doctors have concluded that long term exposure to chemicals found in relaxers and hair dyes are responsible for her serious condition. Salon workers, who frequently perform chemical services for their clients, are also greatly at risk.

61

Short term, occupational exposure to toxic chemicals may cause:[20]

- headaches, nausea and vomiting

- loss of balance

- slurred and slow speech

- mood changes

- hallucinations

- drowsiness

- dizziness

- dermatitis

Long-term occupational exposure to toxic fumes found in salons may result in:[21]

- short term memory loss

- concentration problems

- muscle spasms and motor problems

- peripheral nerve damage

If you suffer from any of these conditions, you should consult with your doctor or seek the attention of a medical professional immediately.

* * * *

We have all had our fair share of bad experiences with relaxers. But many of us never blame our perm or the manufacturer for our hair woes. Instead, we blame ourselves, stress, genetics, our stylist, or any other excuse that we can think of to explain our breakage, hair loss, and/or thinning edges. The time has come, however, for black women to stop making excuses and start doing their homework. Relaxers not only leave us with hair that is dry, brittle, and over-processed -- but these chemicals may affect and harm our long-term health. Like millions of smokers, black women may not learn the truth about perms until it is much too late.

The good news is that there are plenty of beautiful styles for those of us with kinky hair. If you think going natural means spending your Saturday mornings in the kitchen with a jar of TCB grease and a pressing comb, then you have a lot to learn. Many natural styles don't require you to straighten your hair at all. But if you love wearing your hair in a wrap, then ceramic flat irons and ionic blow dryers can give you relaxer results without exposing you to the toxicity of a chemical relaxer. Today, being natural means having options, whether you chose to care for your hair at home or with the help of a stylist.

Are you feeling empowered? You should be. You now know the big secrets that the manufacturers of all of those seductively named products promising 'better' hair do not want you to know. Despite what they claim on the outside of the box, these treatments are seriously dangerous and damaging to your hair. So what are you going to do, continue to use that stuff? OR, will you throw it all away and learn how to care for your hair naturally? I knew you'd make the right decision! As you continue along this journey, you'll soon see why taking the plunge is easier than you think and why your decision to go natural will be one that you will not only never regret…but revel in.

Key Points to Remember

- A relaxer is a chemical process that loosens the hair's natural curl pattern.

- Relaxers strip away the hair's natural moisture, leaving it dry, brittle, and prone to breakage.

- Relaxers are often sold to the public without prior FDA approval.

- The long term effects of using relaxers remain dangerous and *63* unknown.

Chapter 7

In the Pursuit of Nappiness

When I made the decision to go natural, I didn't know the first thing about caring for my kinky tresses. Like so many transitioners before me, I had hundreds of questions and literally nowhere to turn for answers. To say the least, I was lost and confused. Most of the books I read contained very few details about routine care and maintenance and pictured models from the *1980s* wearing styles we wouldn't be caught dead in today. Can you say hair disaster?

Luckily, I met women riding the subway, in the grocery store, and on the Internet with beautiful *modern* natural styles who were kind enough to give me the low down. As I continued to do more research, I quickly became an expert on the subject -- and my friends and colleagues started asking me for transitioning tips, product picks, and styling recommendations. After speaking with hundreds of women about the fears and anxieties that come with going natural, I've compiled a list of the most popular questions to help you get started on your life-changing journey.

What is transitioning?

Transitioning is when you say adios to all those nasty chemicals that broke off your hair and stole so much of your precious time and money. The amount of time it takes to transition from relaxed to natural hair is based entirely on personal preference. Some naturals opt to cut their relaxed ends off gradually -- while others forego the transition process entirely.

How long should I transition for?

If you've been paying attention and taking notes, then the duration of your transition is entirely up to you. Remember, the image of the awful birds nest. Just in case you missed it, here's a tip for you: Don't take your braids out and wash your hair without detangling it first. Again, my job is to keep you from making the same mistakes that I did.

Women who choose to forego the transition process entirely will typically cut their hair into a Teeny Weeny Afro (TWA). A TWA is chic and sexy and gives the wearer tremendous flexibility. "Not only is the style great and totally liberating," says Candace from Atlanta, "but it looks good ALL the time." A TWA is not just for those with small oval faces and perfectly symmetrical features. Women with faces of all shapes and sizes can wear this sophisticated hairstyle. Depending on the look you are trying to achieve, a TWA can be modern and funky or soft and feminine.

Many transitioners will let a barber (or a close friend) perform *The Big Chop*, while others are brave enough to take matters into their own hands. If you decide to do *The Big Chop* at home, make sure that your hair is wet -- so that you can see the point where the relaxed and natural textures meet. You'll also want to be careful and use scissors that are specifically designed for cutting hair. Using plain, old, everyday scissors may leave you with split ends and could end up damaging your natural texture. These are just a few tips to keep in mind to help you get started on the right track.

66 If you have a barber cut off your relaxed ends, be very specific about how you would like your hair to look in terms of length, shape, etc. Note: you should avoid asking for a "*line up*," which is barbershop terminology for a fade. For a softer, more feminine style, ask your barber to cut you hair even all the way around using at least a one-half inch guard. It might also be helpful to bring pictures or magazine photos along to give him or her an idea of what you have in mind. Don't be shy. Make your intentions clear before the scissors hit the hair. Got it? Good.

If I had to do it all over again, I would have definitely gone the TWA route. The great thing about this style it that you get the chance to watch your natural mane come into its own and experiment with it at different lengths. Plus, many naturals find that their hair grows faster once they chop off their relaxed ends.

If your goal, however, is to transition for as long as possible, it's important to settle on styles and a routine that involve a minimum amount of manipulation. Since your natural texture is thicker and stronger than your relaxed ends, your hair will be more prone to breakage where the two textures meet. To avoid looking like Jagged Edge, you'll want to choose styles that can be worn for several days and do not require frequent brushing or combing. Remember, your new hair mantra is *Easy Hair Care.*

What styles are suitable for transitioning?

To keep your hair from breaking while growing out your perm, natural-hair-care expert Syretta Scott, whose A-list clientel includes Jill Scott, Les Nubians, Kindred, and Floetry suggests wearing protective styles - like braids, flat twists, and china bumps - which do not require much combing or brushing. If you prefer looser styles, Scott reccomends going for textured do's like roller sets, straw sets or two-strand twists, which can help minimize the difference in texture between your natural roots and relaxed ends.

Some naturals also opt to transition by straightening their new growth using a flat iron and/or a pressing comb. Using a heated styling appliance will help you to achieve one uniform texture and may minimize breakage – but it can also permanently straighten your natural texture if done too frequently. Wearing a wig or hair extensions is also an option to consider if you prefer to cut your relaxed ends off gradually. While a wig may be convenient occasionally, you shouldn't become dependent on this crutch (as I did) – which will ultimately make the transitioning process more difficult.

67

Wearing a wig is also not the best thing for your newly, natural hair since it obviously keeps it covered. You'll ultimately want to settle on a style that allows you to nurture your new growth, while minimizing the stress on the fragile sections of your hair. So, I strongly suggest finding protetective styles that you like, experimenting with them, and letting the new hair hang out!

While transitioning, it's extremely important to keep your hair and scalp moisturized. "If you allow your hair to become dry and brittle, you'll start to see a lot of breakage," says Scott. Although certain styles can be worn to keep your strands from breaking, it can be extremely difficult to keep your natural hair well conditioned. At the very least, you should be deep conditioning your hair at least once a week to make sure your hair stays soft and manageable.

Frequent trims (every four to six weeks) are also essential. It's a common misconception that natural hair doesn't need to be trimmed. This is absolutely, 100% untrue! If left untreated, split ends will travel further up the hair shaft. Since split ends can't be repaired, your natural hair will be left permanently damaged and will most likely need to be cut off. So, take my advice and get your ends clipped regularly. You don't want to do another *Big Chop*, do you?

What will my family and friends think?

We typically look to our family and friends for support when making major life decisions. Transitioning from relaxed to natural hair is no exception. While your family and friends may love you, they may not completely agree with or support your natural hair preference. But please, don't be discouraged! In many instances, they're just misinformed and lack a basic understanding about the dangers of relaxers. They'll soon see how thick and healthy your natural hair is/becomes and realize that breakage and thinning edges are now a distant memory. In time, you may even find yourself becoming a natural celebrity to loved ones who continue to fight a never-ending battle with over-processed hair and disappearing edges.

Nancy Redd, one of my good friends from college, gave me great advice for dealing with family and friends when I made the decision to go natural. Despite the many compliments Nancy receives on her hair, which is now bra strap length, her mother, her aunts, and many of her friends were strongly opposed to the idea of her wearing her hair natural. She recalls arguing constantly with her mother about relaxing her hair before starting her freshmen year at Harvard. "I know it sounds ridiculous, but my mom is Southern and old school," explains Redd. "She just thought it was plain wrong to send her daughter off to the Ivy League without a relaxer."

After months of fighting, Nancy and her mom reached a compromise -- a press and curl. "It's ironic," says Nancy, "because here we are years later and everyone who insisted I get a perm before leaving for school is

68

now wearing their hair natural!" To catch a glimpse of her head-turning locks, check out the former Miss Virginia's website and latest book, Body Drama, at www.nancyredd.com.

If you're in a relationship, the thought of your significant other not liking your hair can also be challenging as you choose to make this transition. When I first started dating my boyfriend, I didn't want to ruin a good relationship over a bad hairstyle. In fact, part of the reason I wore a wig for almost two years is because I feared my boyfriend would break up with me over my natural hair. Although it did take some getting used to, he eventually grew to love my Afro puff.

Fortunately, after dating for three years, we managed to get past the superficial things and learned to accept each other for who we really were. But, I won't lie to you. There are definitely men out there who will drop you the minute you take out your extensions or put on an extra ten pounds. Honestly, these are not the type of men who are capable of building long-lasting relationships -- nor the type who will stand by your side for a lifetime. Just ask yourself, if a man dumps you over a hairstyle, do you really want to be with him in the first place?

69

What can I expect when I transition?

The transition period can be an emotional rollercoaster. One day you're up and filled with excitement and the next day you're down and overwhelmed by feelings of fear, frustration, and confusion. Every person's experience will be unique. You may also struggle with the idea of wanting to relax or texturize your hair. This is perfectly normal. It took Michelle from Los Angeles three tries before she finally succeeded in going natural. Now that she's successfully made the transition, she wishes she had never given in to the temptation of relaxing her hair when times got rough. She says, "I should have been stronger. . . It only took twenty minutes to destroy all that I had accomplished in five months."

In the course of writing this book, I've spoken to many women who, like Michelle, made a rash decision they would later come to regret in a single moment of weakness. Not only were they disappointed with themselves, they were faced with the fact that they had to begin the entire process all over again from scratch, when they had been so close to reaching their natural goal.

Before you give up and schedule an appointment for a touch-up, here are a few tips to keep you on course: First off, relax. Take a deep breath. Now, repeat these phrases. *My hair will be fine. I will look great. Patience is a virtue.* Yes, the transition period can be difficult. But there is no greater feeling than coming to the realization that your natural hair is beautiful. Try to keep this in mind when you're filled with doubt or worry.

I would also recommend finding a natural buddy who can help you stay focused and reach your ultimate goal. This person can be someone who is already natural or who is also in the process of going natural. I would have never made it through the transition if it weren't for my best friend, Cassie. When times got rough and I couldn't run a comb through my hair, Cassie was there to tell me to put down the jar of Affirm and stay strong!

Collecting magazine photos of natural hairstyles can also provide you with a much needed lift -- but remember, many of these models have weaves or have had their hair professionally done. While transitioning, I would tape pictures of women wearing beautiful natural styles to my bathroom mirror. Whenever I felt like giving up, I just glanced at my natural wall of glory and I'd suddenly feel really good about my decision to let go of relaxers for good. Websites like www.nappturality.com also offer chat rooms and message boards for women who have been through or are going through the same experience. This type of support can be a great source of inspiration when you're feeling down. Finally, you can search online for natural support groups that meet in your area or even consider forming your own.

The transition period is by far the most difficult phase of your natural journey. Fortunately, I'm here to guide you to your natural destination. Don't let a friend, your stylist's sarcastic comments, or one bad hair day stand in the way of you reaching your ultimate, natural goal. Just continue to stay focused and don't give up. I promise you, this is one decision you'll never regret.

Transitioning Tips

Here are ten tips from the pros to make your transition easier:

1. **Be patient.** Transitioning from relaxed to natural hair takes time -- but having patience will make the journey all the more enjoyable. This is the time when you should be getting to know your natural texture, which means you should be having fun and experimenting with different styles and products.

2. **Use a Moisturizing Shampoo.** A good moisturizing shampoo like Nature's Gate Aloe Vera Moisturizing Shampoo will gently cleanse your hair without stripping it dry of its natural oils. You should also be washing your hair at least every seven to ten days to keep your natural hair soft and moisturized.

3. **Deep Condition, Deep Condition, Deep Condition!** As your relaxer grows out, your new growth may start to feel dry and hard. Keep your hair on the right track by using a deep conditioner after every shampoo such as Aveda Damage Remedy Intensive Restructuring Treatment.

   71

4. **Use a Good Detangler.** A good detangler can make it easier to comb through relaxed and natural hair. For smooth and gentle detangling, apply Elucene's Silk Hydrating Elixir to damp hair and always remember to use a wide-tooth comb to work through any knots or tangles.

5. **Hot Oil Treatments.** Pump up the moisture with monthly hot oil treatments made with Vitamin E and olive oil. This all natural formula will help to repair the hair's cuticle and maintain your strands' natural moisture balance.

6. **Go Light.** Go for styling products made with natural oils instead of heavy pomades, gels, and waxes. Light oils are not only easily absorbed by the hair and scalp, but they help to nurture and condition your natural hair as it grows.

7. ***Get Regular Trims.*** Trimming your ends can make combing your hair easier. Some naturals even report that cutting off 1-2" of their relaxed ends helped their natural hair to grow faster.

8. ***Put the Brakes on Color.*** If you can help it, avoid coloring your hair while transitioning. There is no point in using harsh chemicals on already fragile hair. Hair extensions with highlights are a great alternative and can give you a hint of color without the damage.

9. ***Minimize Heat Styling.*** Avoid going overboard with pressing and flat ironing. Too much heat can reduce the hair's elasticity and cause breakage.

10. ***Accessorize.*** If you're bored with your transition style, try barrettes, scarves, or a headband for a different look. Earrings are also a great way to give your do a lift. Try wearing large silver hoops or long, dangling earrings for a style that is sexy and modern -- or go for a sophisticated look and accessorize with a pair of pearl or rhinestone studs.

Transition Styles

In the Pursuit of Nappiness

Twist Outs

The beauty of the twist out is that your hair looks terrific, even if it's out of place. This style looks great on Lenore, who prefered wearing her hair loose during the transitional process. This carefree do is one of my favorites and can be achieved by setting the hair on flexi rods and sitting under the dryer for an hour.

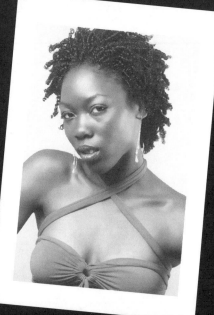

74

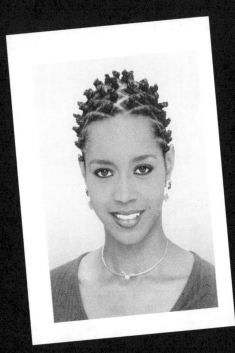

China Bumps

Diamond's look is fresh and modern. This style is for those who want to look great without spending a ton of time on upkeep and maintenance. Get the look by braiding your hair in sections and then wrapping each braid around itself. This do will last up to two weeks if you wear your scarf at night and spray your hair with oil sheen every few days.

75

Braids

Getting braids is a great way to keep breakage at bay and give your hair a rest from harsh chemicals and heat styling. "Not only are they extremely convenient, but your styling options are unlimited," says master braider Lynette "Pinky" Johnson of Propserity Hair and Beauty Salon in Baltimore, MD. Braids can be pulled back into a bun for work, worn down on the weekends, or pinned up for special occasions. If you're considering braids as an option, be sure to consult with an experienced stylist and explain to them that you're in the transition process.

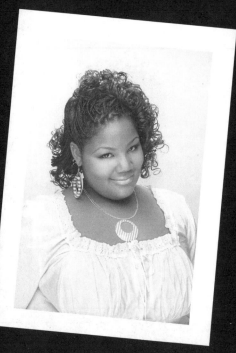

76

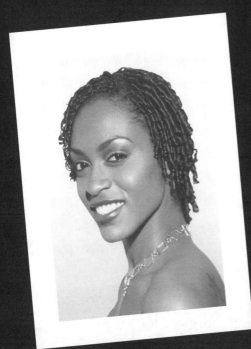

Straw Set

This straw set looks great on Andaye who wanted a style that could take her from the office to happy hour at her favorite after work spot. Andaye's look can be achieved by washing the hair, placing it on straws, and then letting it dry. This transition style doesn't require any heat in between trips to the salon and can last for up to three weeks. For curls that are soft and defined, try using Black Earth Products' Crinkles & Curls Styling Lotion to give the hair a smooth and shiny finish.

77

Wrap

For those who like to wear their hair straight, the wrap is always an option. To keep this style in tact and looking good, you'll need to straighten your new growth regularly with a blow dryer and flat iron. But, be careful -- straightening your hair too frequently can damage your natural texture.

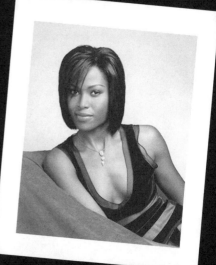

78

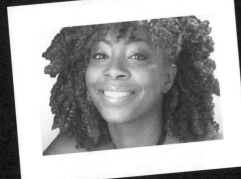

Curly Weave

Transitioning with a weave can help to minimize manipulation, while stimulating natural hair growth. Plus, with the variety of textures and colors to choose from, unbelievably natural looks are easily attainable.

79

Wigs

Wigs are great for transitioning. There are many styles and colors to choose from. The best part is that you can find a good wig for less than $25 and they can last from six months to up to a year. If the game plan is to wear a wig for a week or longer, your best bet is to wear cornrows underneath a wig cap to keep from having to comb your hair everyday. But remember, this is supposed to be a temporary solution. You do not want to become too attached to wigs and then be afraid to make the transition to natural hair, if that is the goal.

80

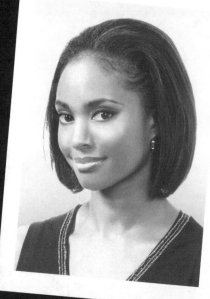

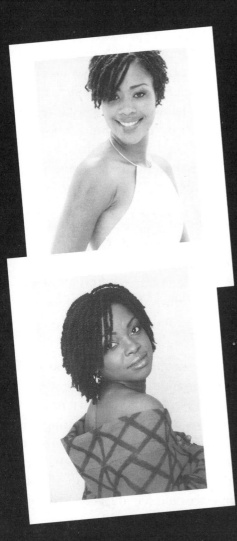

Two-Strand Twist Extensions

This transition style is great for those who want the look of natural hair without waiting. Plus, this look will give your hair a much needed break from brushing and combing and help keep you on track to a smooth transition.

Transitioning with a Weave

If you're frustrated with having to deal with two textures or just looking to experiment with a new style, extensions may offer the perfect solution. Weaves are a great protective style for transitioning and may even help to stimulate natural hair growth. Plus, with the variety of textures and colors to choose from, unbelievably natural looks are easily attainable. "Many of my clients are transitioning to extensions because they want flexibility when it comes to styling," says superstar stylist Kimberly Kimble, whose celebrity clients include Beyoncé Knowles, Gabrielle Union, Kerry Washington, and Mary J. Blige. With extensions, "transitioners have a range of options from the layered wrap to the kinky 'fro and everything in between," says Kimble.

Most stylists, specializing in hair extensions, recommend getting a sew-in weave if you are planning on going natural. With the sew-in method, the hair is cornrowed and the extensions are attached to the braids using a heavy weaving thread. "If done correctly, this technique can be far less damaging to your hair than other methods (e.g. fusion or bonding), which require glue or wax," says Kimble.

Although weaves provide you with a way to minimize the hassle of dealing with two textures, it is still important to take care of your own hair while transitioning with extensions. Neglecting your own hair can lead to breakage and damage and defeats the purpose of wearing this protective style. You should also give the same care to your extensions that you would give to your own natural hair. Remember, the better you care for your extensions, the better they'll look and the longer they'll last. Here are some tips for keeping your extensions looking good and your natural hair healthy:

Tip #1 - Invest in Quality Hair. When it comes to hair, you definitely get what you pay for!!! Inexpensive or cheap hair extensions tangle and matte very easily and usually don't last past the first shampooing. If you choose to purchase hair from your local beauty supply store, Kimble recommends going with Hollywood Hair. For high-end extensions that last, Kimble loves Kimble Creations. "You can use the hair over and over again and it never tangles," say Kimble. For the Afro kinky look, try Afro hair by Adorable.

Tip #2 - Wash Frequently. With a weave, you should be shampooing and conditioning your hair at least once a week. To minimize tangles, brush the hair before shampooing and wash your hair while standing up in the shower. When shampooing, rinse well between tracks to eliminate any residue. For best results, use a gentle moisturizing shampoo like Kimble Hair Care Systems Untangle the Shampoo and finish with Kimble Hair Care Systems Untangle the Conditioner to keep your natural hair moisturized.

Tip #3 – Dry Hair Thoroughly. Make sure you always dry your hair thoroughly *immediately* after washing it to prevent mildew or a foul odor from developing.

Tip #4 - Keep Your Hair Moisturized. Most women with weaves suffer from damage and hair breakage when they neglect their own hair. To prevent this from happening, apply a light oil like Kemy Oil or Kimble Replenish Oil Drops to your cornrows every two to three days to help keep your natural hair moist and conditioned. Hair extensions should also be oiled every few days, to prevent shedding and breakage. Even though you have extensions, they still need to be moisturized since they are not receiving the benefits of the scalp's natural oils. For problems with dry itchy scalp, try massaging your head with carrot oil or Sulfur 8 Light.

Tip #5 - 2 Months Max. "A sew-in weave should never be left in longer than two months. Leaving extensions in for longer than eight weeks can lead to breakage and matting. Kimble also recommends letting a stylist

Tip #6 - Use Good Products. Using good products will help to eliminate build-up and keep your natural hair as well as the extensions soft and conditioned. Also, keep your product usage to a minimum. Using too many styling aids can give the hair a stringy, greasy look and leave your extensions looking limp and lifeless.

Tip #7 – Never Use a Comb. Use a vent or paddle wig brush instead of a comb to detangle your extensions. Remember, always brush your hair in a downward motion, starting near the ends --gently working your way up to the roots.

Tip # 8 – Avoid/Minimize Heat. Heat is one of your extensions' worse enemies. The more you use it, the shorter your extensions will last. Be extra careful when blow-drying and curling your weave, because burnt hair can't be repaired.

Tip #9 –Never sleep on wet hair. Always make sure your hair is *completely* dry before going to bed to avoid waking up with a bird's nest. It's also a good idea to wrap your hair or sleep with a satin bonnet to help your extensions stay shiny.

84

Tip #10 – Take a Break. If you notice that your hair or hairline has been damaged when you take down your extensions, wait at least four to six weeks before getting another weave put in. While extensions can be a great transition style, if not properly cared for, they can pull the hair out, and may cause hair thinning and leave you with a few bald spots.

Tip #11 – Get a Touch Up. Long heavy extensions can sometimes put pressure on the scalp and cause the hair to fall out. To keep your natural hair looking healthy, see a professional stylist at least once a month to have your extensions retightened and touched up.

Tip #12 – Go Natural!!! The downside to transitioning with a weave is not learning how to care for your natural hair as it grows. If you're using your extensions as a crutch and are scared about the reactions others may have to your natural hair, let go and embrace your natural texture. The sooner you embrace your natural tresses, the better.

How Long Should I Transition For?

There are many factors to take into account when you are deciding to do *The Big Chop*. Here is a little quiz you can take to determine whether to go the TWA route or stick things out for the long haul. Add up the numbers to find out, which option suits you best. Note: your results don't mean you HAVE to transition a certain way; it's just simply a guide for what you can do.

1. **Is your relaxed hair damaged?** *(split ends, breakage, tangly, limp, rough, extra dry?)*

   Yes (20)

   No (10)

2. **How much time are you willing to devote to learn about styling the two textures?**

   As much as necessary (5)

   A fair amount (10)

   A little (15)

   None (20)

3. **How skilled are you at styling your own hair?**

   Very Skilled (5)

   Skilled (10)

   Okay (15)

   Not Skilled (20)

4. **How long do you want to keep your relaxed length?**

   For as long as possible (5)

   For a little while (10)

   Not long (15)

   Cut it off now! (61)

* * * *

Your score: **60+ Points**
Grab a friend and get the scissors because...you're in for "**The Big Chop**"

Your best bet is to do *The Big Chop* sooner rather than later. Starting your natural journey wearing a TWA can be a wonderful thing and will give you plenty of opportunities to experiment with your natural hair as it grows. Plus, this style is super-convenient, which means you don't have to worry about breakage or holding onto your pitiful relaxed ends.

* * * *

Your score: **45 - 60 points**
You're in for the "**Short Transition**"

It looks like you could be in for a short transition (e.g. four to six months). Go for fuss-free styles that require minimal manipulation. If you have skills when it comes to styling, you may be able to get away with a straw or roller set. Flat twists and two-strand twists (extensions or natural) are also options, which can help to minimize the difference between the two textures and get you through this transitional period. If you weren't blessed with skills when it comes to doing your own hair, then consider transitioning with braids or extensions. If your relaxed hair is already damaged, then you should probably just take the plunge and do *The Big Chop* since breakage is almost inevitable. If your hair is healthy, keep in mind that you'll still need to trim your ends regularly to prevent breakage and split ends.

86

* * * *

Your score: **Less than 45 points**
Hold on to your hair... you can execute the "**Long Transition**"

Based on your responses, you may be in for a long transition (e.g. eight to twelve months). Although a small minority of women manage to transition for over a year, many find themselves wishing they had done *The Big Chop* sooner. Note, transitioning for longer than a year may prove counterproductive to your hair's condition. If you're still struggling with whether to get rid of your relaxed ends, please send me an email or give me a call. I'm definitely here to help and offer my support. In the meantime, continue to follow your regular hair-care regimen to ensure that your natural tresses stay healthy and strong.

Key Points to Remember

- Transitioning doesn't have to be difficult - but it requires a great deal of patience.

- The length of time it takes to transition out of your relaxer is a matter of personal preference.

- When transitioning, protective styles should be worn to minimize breakage.

- Keeping your hair and scalp moisturized during the transition phase is extremely important.

- Don't be discouraged if your friends, family, and/or significant other do not support your decision to go natural.

- In your moment of weakness, stay strong and remember how far you have come.

87

Chapter 8

Caring for Your Natural Hair

So you've finally done *The Big Chop*. Congratulations! Now you're dying to rock a fly twist-out with your big silver hoop earrings. Well, *be patient*. Healthy, beautiful, natural hair can be yours without a ton of fuss, *if* you take the time to master the fundamentals of caring for your tresses. So, ladies, let your new mantra be, *"Know Thine Hair."* Your comb coils and flat twists will look ten times better if you shampoo and condition your hair properly, avoid certain products, and learn which styling tools to use to keep your hair looking and feeling its best.

Unconditional Love

The first rule of natural hair is this: *Love Your Hair Unconditionally*. For me, this meant accepting the fact that my hair was not naturally wavy like Mariah Carey's and didn't have major shine like Alicia Keys'. I know my hair may look great in person – but trust me, without any hair products, I look more like Frederick Douglas than I'll ever want to admit! You'll soon discover your own hair eccentricities as well.

With a little patience and a lot of experimentation, you'll find it is easy to groom and care for your natural hair. The hardest part is simply letting go of your preconceived notions about beauty and "your European standards of neatness," says master locktician and natural hair stylist Thierry Baptiste, of Brunette Salon in Indianapolis. Although everyone's hair texture is different, here are some common characteristics that make our natural hair unique:

Uniform Texture. Due to our mixed ancestry, hair textures among black women range from tightly curled to ruler-straight and everything in between. Even on a single head, hair textures and types can vary widely. If you are in the midst of transitioning or if you're already natural, you may notice that the curls along your hairline are loose and wavy, but tight and kinky around the nape of your neck or the crown of your head. Learning to deal with different textures may seem difficult at first -- but you'll quickly learn which styles, techniques, and products work best for your hair type. When it comes to natural hair, Baptiste tells his clients not to obsess over "making sure that every hair is in place, but just to merely let their natural hair be." So, instead of trying to have each hair on your head be uniform, embrace the differences in texture and type and allow your natural style to highlight all the wonderful nuances of your kinky mane.

Shine. Unlike relaxed hair, which tends to have a sheen, the surface of natural hair is uneven and doesn't reflect light well. For this reason, your focus is better spent on having "healthy" natural hair instead of "shiny" natural hair. Just remember, with natural hair, less is more. You'll want to avoid thick and greasy pomades, which promise to deliver moisture and shine. These products often just coat the hair and leave your strands looking dull and lifeless. Your best bet is to stick with natural moisturizers such as jojoba, coconut, and olive oil. These natural emollients work great on natural hair and help give it a healthy glow.

Shrinkage. Natural hair is extremely curly and can shrink anywhere from ten to eighty percent of its actual length. Curly hair is also prone to shrinkage due to its structure, which causes it to bend, twist, and turn. There are many non-chemical alternatives for naturals who would like to stretch out and straighten their curls. Banding, twist outs, and roller sets are all styles that can help the hair to show its length -- and are described in greater detail later in the book.

Moisture. Natural hair loves water! When you were relaxed, water, humidity, and sweat were your hair's worst enemies. But natural hair actually thrives on moisture. Black hair tends to be dry and requires extra moisture and conditioning since, as mentioned before, the oils produced by the scalp don't travel down the curved follicle or curled hair as freely as they would in straight hair. To keep the hair soft and moist, try misting your hair with water every two to three days. Drinking eight to ten glasses of water per day will also help to keep your strands healthy and strong (and is great for the skin and the rest of the body too).

Delicate. Because of its texture and appearance, there is a common misconception that kinky hair is strong and can withstand more stress and abuse than white hair. In reality, black hair is extremely delicate and must be handled gently and with care.

Simply put, natural hair requires a lot of TLC. Once you learn to accept your hair for what it is and to love it, despite what it does and does not do, you'll be well on your way to reaching your natural hair goals.

Natural Hair Care Basics

It's a common misconception that natural hair requires no maintenance. Au contraire! Regular maintenance is essential to making sure that your hair stays healthy and looking good. Keeping your hair clean and well conditioned is an absolute must. Trimming your ends is also necessary to prevent split ends, tangles, and breakage. But, you already know this from your experiences with a relaxer, so you're off to a great start. Here are just a few additional tips from some top stylists to keep in mind:

Shampooing

I can remember washing my natural hair for the first time like it was yesterday. When I stepped into the shower, I ran my fingers through my tight curls and felt my real hair texture, something I had not experienced in close to twenty years. Although I had less than one inch of hair then, my hair now hangs down past my shoulders. I've learned from experience *91* that the key to beautiful hair is a clean and healthy scalp.

Healthy hair care begins with washing and conditioning the hair at least once a week to remove any dirt and product build-up on the scalp. If you wash your hair more frequently, there is no need to shampoo your hair twice on one occasion. One good lathering should be enough to clean your scalp without stripping away the hair's natural oils in the process.

Washing your natural hair is almost the same as washing your relaxed hair, with the exception of a few small differences. First, you'll want to use a shampoo rich in moisturizers and emollients. Your choice of shampoo will depend primarily on your hair type. If you hair is oily, a mild shampoo like Jason Natural's 84% Pure Aloe Vera Shampoo Super Shine Shampoo works well, says Natasha Jackson owner of Na'Klectic Natural Hair Gallery in Baltimore, MD. For dry hair, you may consider adding a drop of jojoba oil to your regular shampoo to give your hair extra moisture. Camille Reed of Noire Designs in Washington, D.C. also recommends sleeping with olive oil on your hair the night before you shampoo for added shine and softness.

Many people, when washing their hair, make the mistake of creating lots of suds and then roughly scrubbing the hair and scalp. They think this is helping to thoroughly clean their mane, but in actuality, they just may find themselves with a bird's nest on top of their head! The more tangled the hair becomes, the harder it is to really rinse out all the shampoo and conditioner. So, please use restraint and be gentle when washing your hair.

Although natural hair can be washed daily, washing your hair too frequently can cause your tresses to become dry and brittle. Since black hair tends to be dry to begin with, this often leads to further problems with split ends and breakage. In between shampoos, it is a good idea to rinse your hair with water daily. If you prefer not to rinse daily, at least mist your hair with water every two to three days to help keep your strands soft and moisturized.

No-Pooing (Conditioner Washes)

If you think your shampoo is causing your hair to feel dry and brittle, you should switch to conditioner washes, also known as no-pooing. I know it sounds silly -- but it's good for you. Many shampoos contain harsh detergents, which strip the hair of its natural oils causing it to become dry and brittle. Instead of using regular shampoos, some naturals use a mild conditioner to remove dirt and impurities that have built up on the scalp. Many women who no-poo, find that their hair is softer, easier to comb, and requires fewer products compared to when they wash their hair using regular shampoo. On the other hand, conditioner washes may not work well if your hair is naturally oily or if you use styling products frequently.

If you switch to conditioner washes, you should no-poo at least once a week, or as often as you did when you washed your hair with regular shampoo. Depending on your hair type, it may not be necessary to use additional conditioner after no-pooing. For best results, try using Pantene Hydrating Curls or Avalon Organic's Awapuhi Mango Moisturizing Conditioner.

Clarifying

If your hair lacks luster or appears duller than usual, then you may be suffering from *product build-up*. In this case, try using a clarifying shampoo, which will help to eliminate the residue from gels, mousses, pomades, and other products that collect on your scalp with regular use. To prevent the hair from drying out, a clarifying shampoo should be used no more than once a month. One of my favorite clarifying shampoos is Suave Daily Clarifying Shampoo (*note this product should not be used daily*) and can be found at your local drug store or pharmacy. Rinsing the hair with one part apple cider vinegar and one part water is also a good, all natural substitute for commercial, clarifying shampoos. An added bonus to this alternative solution: you'll be doing your part for the environment by not buying products that come in plastic bottles, with so much unnecessary packaging. What could be better, a formula that's cheaper, gentler, all natural – and environmentally friendly!

Conditioning

It's always advisable to use a conditioner after shampooing your hair to replenish its natural oils. Conditioners can add shine, reduce tangles, and help repair damaged hair. Since the ends are the oldest part of your hair, be sure to focus on applying the conditioner to this section to protect against breakage and damage. In order to ensure even distribution of the product, I always make it a point to run a large-tooth comb through my hair before rinsing out any conditioner. If you're using a regular conditioner, be sure to let it sit on your hair for approximately two to three minutes. Giving your hair extra time to absorb the product will leave your hair soft and shiny.

For best results, rinse thoroughly with cold water to eliminate all traces of shampoo and conditioner from your hair and scalp. "A cold water rinse causes the cuticle to lay flat and gives the hair an extra shine," says celebrity hair artist Nedjetti of Hair by Nedjetti. For dry hair, Nedjetti recommends a moisturizing or intensive conditioner like Therapeutics RX; for oily hair, a conditioner like Quenching Conditioner by Blended Beauty should get the job done.

Deep conditioning is particularly important since kinky hair tends to be dry. Environmental factors, chemical treatments, and heat styling can also cause our hair to look dull and lifeless. Using a deep conditioner once every two weeks will help to counteract this damage and restore shine and manageability to your tresses.

For best results, cover your hair with a plastic cap and sit under a dryer for thirty minutes in order to allow the deep conditioner to penetrate the hair shaft. But be careful! Using a deep conditioner too often can leave your hair weak and damaged. Frequent use of protein-based, deep conditioners can cause the hair to become dry and brittle and over-use of moisturizing or oil-based deep conditioners can result in your hair appearing limp and lifeless. "For an intense moisturizing experience, try adding a half of a cup of mashed avocado or a tablespoon of olive oil to your deep conditoning treatments," says stylist Tinesha Deadwiley of Lockstar Salon in Charlotte, NC. A dollop of mayonaise will also do the trick. In between treatments, Deadwiley advises doing a hot oil treatment. This can help repair the damage that neglect and constant styling can cause. It is also a great way to enhance the natural shine and texture of your hair.

Detangling

In order to make combing easier and manageable, once you have completely rinsed out your conditioner, apply a detangling conditioner, such as Paul Mitchell's The Detangler, to the hair while it is still damp. Next, run a wide-tooth comb through your hair several times to remove any knots and tangles. Be patient and gentle as you detangle the hair until you can comb through it easily. If you ever come across a difficult knot, use your fingers to remove the tangle in order to prevent breakage or damage. If you hair is longer than five inches, you may find it easier to part your hair into four sections and tackle one section at a time. To make detangling easier, keep a spray bottle close by and spritz as necessary to prevent your hair from drying out.

With a relaxer, it is easy to run a comb through your tresses from roots to ends to undo any knots and tangles. With natural hair, the process is almost the exact opposite. Instead of combing from top to bottom, you'll want to start by detangling your ends first and working your way gradually up to the roots -- in a slow and steady motion.

With kinky hair, each curl represents a delicate point along the hair shaft. If you comb too quickly or in the wrong direction, you can literally hear the sound of your hair breaking. "This is why little black girls cry when they get their hair combed," says mane pro Symone Hilton of Natural Trendsetters Salon in Miami, FL. "It's not that they're tenderheaded. It's just that so many black mothers don't understand how to properly comb and care for their daughter's hair." Detangling curly or kinky texture hair is best done with a large, wide-tooth comb, while the hair is still damp. For wavy and straighter textures, a paddle brush is recommended.

I personally find it easier to detangle my hair with a Denman Brush once I have combed through it once or twice with a wide-tooth comb. *95* A Denman Brush is made with smooth nylon pins set into an anti-static rubber pad and can be purchased at your local beauty supply store. I swear completely by the D4 Denman Brush, although many other models are available. In my opinion, this brush is one of the best styling tools for untangling naturally curly tresses and removing shed hair without damaging your strands.

Hot Oil Treatments

Treating your tresses to a hot oil treatment can help to repair your hair's cuticles and restore shine and softness within a matter of minutes. A hot oil treatment goes far beyond basic conditioning. It also helps to reduce frizz, control split ends, and improve the overall texture and strength of your hair in the long run. With just plain ole olive oil you can get dramatic results that leave your hair twice as strong and shiny after just one use. This weekly, pre-shampoo conditioning treatment rinses out easily and adds moisture and vitality to brittle hair strands. To use, break open a vitamin E capsule and add the contents to a one-half cup of olive oil, and warm in the microwave for thirty seconds. Before shampooing, massage the treatment onto wet hair. Leave on for up to three minutes. Rinse hair and scalp thoroughly. Shampoo as usual. Apply weekly or more often, as needed.

Trimming

Natural hair should be trimmed every two to three months to keep it looking healthy and to prevent split ends. Natural hair that isn't trimmed regularly won't retain moisture well and will ultimately become extremely difficult to comb, says Tonya Reed, master stylist and owner of Uncle Funky's Daughter Hair Salon in Houston, TX. I would strongly recommend making an appointment at a natural-friendly salon at least four times a year to get your ends trimmed – and to receive a second opinion on the health and overall condition of your hair. Although every stylist has their own preferences, Reed recommends trimming the hair while it is damp, if you wear your hair curly most of the time, and trimming the hair when it's dry if you mainly wearing it straight.

Diet

96

Diet also plays an important role in maintaining a head full of healthy, natural hair. Good nutrition not only affects the hair, but also the skin and scalp. Eating foods rich in vitamins and minerals can dramatically improve the health of your hair. Certain vitamins and minerals have also been shown to prevent or reduce hair loss, increase shine and manageability, and maintain the overall condition of already healthy hair. You can easily increase your vitamin intake by eating fresh fruit and vegetables or taking vitamin supplements. Drinking plenty of water will also keep your strands hydrated and supple. It is important to realize that when it comes down to it, the condition of your hair is a reflection of your overall health. Eating properly and taking good care of yourself will keep both hair and body looking and feeling its best.

Vitamins for Healthy Hair

Good nutrition is just as essential to healthy hair growth as it is to your overall health/well-being. Just as your body needs a variety of nutrients in order to function properly, there are several vitamins and minerals that can help to can maximize your hair's growth and potential.

- **Vitamin A** produces healthy sebum in the scalp. Food sources: raw tomatoes, mangos, broccoli, carrots, oranges, fish liver oil, meat, milk, cheese, eggs, spinach, broccoli, cabbage, and carrots.

- **Vitamin B5 (Pantothenic Acid)** prevents graying and hair loss. Food sources: whole grain cereals, Brewer's yeast, organ meats, and egg yolks.

- **Vitamin B6** produces keratin and prevents hair loss. Food sources: whole grain cereals, vegetables, organ meats, egg yolk, and liver.

- **Vitamin C** is important for growth and maintaining healthy hair. Food sources: fresh fruit, such as oranges, grapefruit, kiwi, cantaloupe, pineapple, and dark green vegetables.

- **Vitamin E** enhances scalp circulation. Food sources: cold-pressed vegetable oils, wheat germ oil, soybeans, raw seeds, nuts, dried beans, and leafy green vegetables.

- **Biotin** helps to produce keratin and may also prevent hair loss and greying. Food sources: egg yolks, liver, rice, and Brewer's yeast.

- **Iron** helps to reduce hair loss. Food sources: lean red meat, raisins, eggs, whole grain cereals, and dark green vegetables.

- **Inositol** keeps hair follicles healthy. Food sources: whole grains, liver, and citrus fruits.

WARNING. When starting a new vitamin program, it can take anywhere from two to three months to see a change in your hair's condition. That means patience and consistency are very important. You should also consult with your doctor or preferred health care provider before taking any vitamin supplements, especially if you are currently taking any other medication or have a pre-existing health condition that can affect your medical treatment. Remember, just because they're vitamins doesn't mean they're not dangerous!

Here is some additional advice from the pros on how to help keep your strands looking their best:

- **Mucho Moisture.** "Keeping your hair moisturized, conditioned and trimmed regularly is an absolute must for preventing breakage and minimizing split ends," says celebrity stylist A.J. Johnson of AJES The Salon in Chicago. Since black hair tends to be dry, A.J. loves products that contain natural ingredients and light oils that can be easily absorbed by the hair, and encourages his clients to steer clean of products containing beeswax, lanolin, and petroleum – which merely coat the strands and have a tendency to attract dust and lint.

- **Never comb dry hair.** Always mist your hair with water or apply a small amount of pomade to your tresses to help the comb glide through your locks. Go slowly and if you come across a tangle or knot, try to detangle it with your fingers first before going for a comb. Avoid small combs with sharp teeth, which can tear the hair. Instead, use larger combs with rounded teeth and smooth edges.

- **Don't overbrush.** Forget the old saying about brushing 100 strokes a day! The truth is, over-brushing can lead to breakage. Regular, gentle brushing is okay, but be sure to invest in a brush with firm bristles with rounded ends.

- **Get your beauty sleep.** Sleep wearing a satin scarf or bonnet, or if you prefer to sleep with your head uncovered, purchase a satin pillow case. Wool and cotton strip the hair of its natural oils, leaving it dry, brittle, and prone to breakage. If you live in a cooler climate, protect your hair from wool and cotton hats and scarves by wearing a satin scarf underneath your cap or by purchasing silk-lined winter accessories.

- **Treat your scalp.** Take a few minutes each day to give yourself a scalp massage "This simple practice increases the circulation in the scalp area and promotes healthy oil production," says Jill Scott's go to stylist Syreeta Scott, owner of Duafe Holistic Hair Care Natural Hair Salon in Philidaelphia.

- **Turn off the heat.** Blow dryers and curling irons can cause considerable damage to the hair and, in some cases, can permanently straighten your natural texture. Instead of heat styling, consider natural styles such as braids, twist-outs or a puff, which can be achieved without causing major damage to your hair.

- **Keep your ends protected.** Once your hair reaches shoulder length, the constant friction caused by your hair rubbing against your clothes often results in dryness and breakage. You can avoid this by wearing protective hairstyles, which don't leave your ends exposed, and keeping your ends well condtioned.

- **Choose your stylist wisely.** Choose a hairdresser that you feel comfortable with and who specializes in caring for natural hair. Finding the right stylist is one of the most important steps to developing your personal style and growing beautiful, healthy tresses. A good stylist will be honest with you and take the time to educate you about your hair. To locate a stylist in your area, check out the Salon Directory in the back of the book or on my website at www.thankgodimnatural.com.

99

* * * *

Three years ago, I can remember looking at pictures in *Essence* magazines and being inspired by the pages filled with beautiful twist-outs, chunky Afros, and comb coils. Unfortunately, my hair didn't come close to looking anything like what I saw in those photos. Although my hair was soft and moisturized, it looked dull and lifeless. Wearing a wig for so long had definitely taken its toll on my hair's condition. But once I went completely natural, my hair began to flourish. It was a slow process -- with many ups and downs -- but my hair is now thick and healthy and also ironically, the longest it has ever been. Slowly but surely, things started to make sense and all of the pieces began to fit together. Now, with each day that goes by, I continue to grow stronger and more confident that my hair is beautiful just the way it is.

I have shared with you my best practices to help you keep your natural hair looking healthy and beautiful. The most important thing to remember is to always treat your mane with love. Your hair can never get enough TLC! Whether you take care of your tresses at home or with the help of a professional stylist, natural hair will soon become one of your greatest beauty assets. Mastering the basics is easy - but it will take time and a great deal of patience. Before long, you'll be well on your way to creating beautiful styles that suit your personality, style, and ultimately your sense of self.

110

Key Points to Remember

- Grooming and caring for your natural tresses will be easier if you accept your hair for what it is.

- Keeping your hair clean, conditioned, and well mositurized is essential to achieving a healthy mane.

- Hair should be trimmed at least four to five times a year to prevent split ends, tangles and breakage.

- Eating properly and taking good care of yourself will help keep your hair looking its best.

101

Chapter 9

Get Lock'd Up

Bob Marley is widely credited for bringing reggae music to the masses. But as he did, he probably had no clue that he would be remembered as much for his distinctive locks as for his musical genius. While Rastafarians are often attributed with inventing this hairstyle, the origin of wearing locks can actually be traced as far back as 2500 BC. Once considered taboo, locks have thankfully gained widespread acceptance in today's society and in most professional circles -- giving many of us the freedom to choose this wonderful form of personal expression. We thank you, Bob Marley, not only for the music, but also for your hair. *One Love!*

Deciding to get locks is an extremely personal decision -- and one that is imbued with various meanings for each individual. For Joy, from San Francisco, the choice to grow locks was born out of pure laziness. "I was looking for a style that was versatile enough to take me from sunshine to rain and that would also allow me to sleep in an extra fifteen to twenty minutes in the morning." Michelle, from Washington D.C., made the decision to lock when she reached the point where finally felt comfortable in her own skin. As she puts it, "I never thought I would be strong enough to defy the media and do what was best for me. But once I started wearing them, I knew that I had made the right decision." As you can see, the reasons for selecting this unique style range from the challenges of dealing with the morning lethargy to aesthetic concerns, and everything in between. Like any choice, take some time to reflect on what would work best for you before making up your mind.

Before You Lock

Thanks to innovations in techniques, locks have become a versatile styling option for people of all ages, genders, and different walks of life. Unlike most styles, growing locks requires lots of patience. For most women, however, the decision to start locks isn't an easy one. Celebrity stylist Veronica Sirca, the force behind Lauryn Hill's gorgeous mane, explains, "A woman must be strong and confident enough to accept her natural texture for what it is." Once you do decide to embrace locks, don't second-guess yourself – enjoy them! Remember, nothing has to be permanent with hair and you can always select another style down the line if this one doesn't suit you. Still, give locks a chance – you may surprise yourself and others with the bold new do!

Before taking the plunge, make sure you do your homework and know what you are getting yourself into. Here are a few things to consider before you make this commitment: *How physically active are you? Do you plan to maintain your locks at home or with the help of a locktician? How much time and money are you willing to spend on caring for your hair? What look are you trying to achieve?*

Sirca also discourages anyone from getting locks that has not experienced what it's like to wear their natural hair loose. "Many people who transition from a relaxer straight into locks often feel like they skipped a step," she says. For this reason, Sirca recommends experimenting with different natural styles for at least a year before committing to locks -- to give yourself the chance to fully enjoy (and become accustomed to) your natural tresses.

Something else to keep in mind before selecting this particular style *104* is that your locks will never look absolutely perfect. This is what makes this style so beautiful and unique. Each lock may vary in shape and size. Some hairs may stick out while others stay neatly in place. Your roots may be loose, while your ends are tightly compacted together. All of these characteristics make locks such an amazing and liberating hairstyle. Again, dealing with these imperfections is just one aspect of having locks. If imperfection isn't something your personality can tolerate, perhaps you should reconsider your decision to grow them in the first place.

Starting Locks at Home or with a Professional

Whether you choose to start locks at home or with the help of a professional is simply a matter of personal preference. An experienced locktician can advise you as to what size locks and locking method are appropriate, given the texture and thickness of your hair. During your initial consultation, the stylist may also ask you questions about your lifestyle, grooming regimen, hair history and health – in order to help you achieve optimal results. If you choose to have your locks started by a professional, make sure you ask him/her: *How thick or thin will they be? What products do you use? How often should I get maintenance on them? How do I care for my locks? How much do you charge for starting locks?*

How much do you charge to re-twist them? Knowing the answers to these questions can help you to select a qualified locktician and assist you in determining whether this style is right for you. You'll also want to check out your stylist's locks to make sure they are on point. The condition of your locktician's own hair is typically a great indicator of how skilled they are when it comes to caring for their clients' hair.

If you are considering starting your locks at home, it is often a good idea to play it safe and have a consultation with a professional before embarking upon the do-it-yourself method. The locktician will help you select a technique that fits with your lifestyle and hair type. He or she can also give you initial direction and guidance on this journey. If you start to feel discouraged by your decision to lock, keep in mind that you're not the first person to grow and maintain this style at home. If you find yourself becoming frustrated or discouraged, check out www.mydreadlocks.com, where you can find answers to many of your questions. The website www.nappturality.com is also a great place to meet other women who are locked or are starting the process for the first time.

Locking Methods

Locks can be started in many different ways. Depending on the initial length and texture of your hair and how much time and money you want to spend on maintenance, it may be preferable to start with one method versus another. The method you choose can also have a definite impact on the final shape and texture of your locks. Just make sure you choose a method that suits your hair, your budget and your lifestyle.

Starting with Comb Coils

Comb coils (a/k/a comb twists) are one of the classic techniques that can be used to start locks. Comb coils look great on short hair and are extremely shiny when freshly done. Unfortunately, comb coils don't remain in tact as well as other locking methods and can become frizzy. Frequent re-twisting, at least once every three weeks, is usually a must with comb coils, since they tend to unravel easily, especially after the hair is washed or if it is naturally straight or wavy. Comb coils are also great if your hair is short (1- 3") and tightly coiled. If your hair is longer, Sirca suggests starting with double strand twists.

You can achieve comb coils at home simply by parting your hair into small sections (almost the size of a pencil) and applying a small amount of Aloe Vera gel to the area that is to be twisted. To create coils, gently gather a small section of hair near your scalp with the teeth of a rat-tail comb and begin twisting your hair in a downward motion until you create a spiral-shaped lock. Continue onto the next section and repeat until you have finished your entire head. Be patient, if you're not successful at first. It may take time and practice before you are completely satisfied with the results.

Starting with Palm rolls

Palm rolling is one of the traditional methods for starting locks. In general, this technique is used on longer, tightly coiled texture hair (3-5") to produce locks that are uniform in shape and size. Like comb twists, palm rolls can come undone fairly easily and require frequent maintenance to remain in tact. Although palm rolls can be created with all hair types, this method works best with coarser textures.

You can create palm rolls at home by parting your hair into small sections (almost the size of a pencil) and applying a small amount of Aloe Vera gel to the area that is to be rolled. Once the hair is separated and you have applied the Aloe Vera gel onto the desired lock, place the sectioned hair in between your hands and begin to slowly rub your palms in one direction until a cylindrical coil or spiral lock begins to form. Just think back to when you were a kid and you would rub play dough in between your hands until you created something that resembled a long skinny snake. The technique is pretty much the same here. Continue onto the next section and repeat until you have finished your entire head.

Starting Locks with Two-Strand Twists

Two strand twists are now frequently used to start locks. This popular hairstyle is highly recommended for longer lengths (5"+) and straighter textures. This technique is similar to braiding, except that twists are created using two strands of hair instead of three. As the hair begins to lock, the roots can be tightened using the palm rolling technique. Although it can take up to a month before the hair begins to matte, it gives the wearer some flexibility if they are uncertain about their decision to lock. Two strand twists are also relatively easy to maintain and can be achieved without the assistance of a locktician.

Starting with Braids

Braids can also be used to start locks and work well on all hair types, including straighter textures. Braids are also an option for those with relaxed or naturally straight hair. As far as length is concerned, you'll need approximately ½" of hair to achieve this style. Keep in mind that braids can frizz quickly, but can generally be palm rolled after six months to give a locked appearance. Despite the drawbacks, braids do not unravel easily and can be shampooed more frequently beginning as early as the second week.

Starting with Sisterlocks ®

Sisterlocks are super thin locks created using a crochet like instrument and a patented technique created by Dr. Joanne Cornwell. Sisterlocks give the wearer tremendous flexibility, since they are thin and can be styled *107* in the same fashion as straight hair. The average Sisterlocks wearer has between 300-450 locks in comparison with the average lock-wearer who has between 100-150 locks. This style can be achieved on either relaxed or natural hair, so long as you have at least 1" of unprocessed hair.

Sisterlocks should be retightened every four to six weeks for the first two to three months and then every six to eight weeks once the hair has begun to matte and the locks have settled. Hair that is dense and tightly coiled will lock faster than hair that is soft, fine, wavy, or straight. The Sisterlocks organization also provides training on how to maintain your locks at home once you have reached the six-month mark. You can obtain more information about Sisterlocks or locate a Sisterlocks consultant in your area by visiting www.sisterlocks.com.

Starting with Extensions

Lock extensions are for those women who can't wait to grow their own locks or who need to repair thinning locks. This style is usually created by a locktician and can be achieved using cotton, spiral hair for a full head of extension locks. Extension locks can be expensive -- but this method allows you to forego the months or years of locking and enjoy beautiful locks almost instantly. "The results are stunning and look completely natural if done by a skilled locktician," says Ewanda Wyndella, owner of Happy To Be Nappy Hair Salon in Detroit, MI -- whose clients often marvel at how closely their extensions resemble locks that were grown naturally.

Freeform Locks

The term "freeform" refers to locks that are grown naturally -- without any artificial, outside manipulation. When one thinks of freeform locks, Reggae superstar Bob Marley often comes to mind. One of the most popular ways to start freeform locks is to rub a towel in a circular motion over freshly washed hair until small clusters start to form. Over time, the clusters will start to matte -- eventually producing individual locks. Another way is to start with twists or coils and then simply stop maintaining the hair after it locks. Freeform locks are extremely low-maintenance and do not require re-twisting, palm rolling or tightening of the roots. Besides shampooing, the hair isn't manipulated in any way. Some freeformers, however, separate their locks –in order to prevent them from crawling into one another and forming one large lock.

A Clean Start

The way your hair is parted and sectioned initially will determine the final shape and size of your locks. If you have a preference for locks that are uniform in shape and size, your best bet is to have them started by a professional. The ability to achieve different styles will depend largely on the length and thickness of your locks. With longer locks, you generally have more styling options. Thin ones are also more flexible to work with and can be styled in a variety of ways. If you prefer thin locks, make sure the hair is parted in small sections initially. Likewise, for medium or larger locks, you'll need to work with larger sections of hair. *Note*: if you start with too small of sections, your locks could break off as they grow longer. While small locks are extremely pretty, you'll need to make sure that your roots can provide a strong enough foundation for them as they mature. So, unless you're getting Sisterlocks, your locks should be no smaller in width than a pencil.

Locks should always be started with clean hair. You can start locks with either wet or dry hair -- but damp hair is usually easier to work with when using the palm roll, comb coil, or two-strand twist techniques. Avoid using products that contain beeswax, petroleum, or lanolin. These products provide excellent hold but are extremely difficult to wash out of your hair since they're not water-soluble. Instead, try using Aloe Vera gel for hold and moisture. Fruit of the Earth Aloe Vera Gel is one of the most popular products for starting locks and makes styling and grooming easy. Black Earth Products' Lock It Up is also great for twisting the hair and won't flake the way most gels do.

If you start locks with wet hair, sit under a hood/bonnet dryer set on medium to give them the chance to settle. If your hair unravels easily, you can secure each lock at the root with a metal clip until your hair dries. Once your locks are dry, spray your scalp with natural oil for moisture and shine.

Lock Stages -At-a-Glance

There are three distinct stages of the locking process: the baby phase, the teenage phase, and the mature phase. Although this journey requires a great deal of time and patience, in the long run, the results can be extremely rewarding. Just be sure to take your time and enjoy every moment.

Baby Locks

The name *"baby locks"* can be misleading. Although cute and adorable, baby locks demand an enormous amount of time and attention. Like any newborn, you'll want to treat your baby locks gently and with the utmost care. Depending upon your hair texture and the method you used to start your locks, this phase can last anywhere from one month to over a year.

Maintaining Baby Locks

A common misconception about baby locks is that you can't wash your hair during this phase. This is absolutely false! Sirca suggests waiting at least three to four weeks before shampooing your brand new baby locks to give them the chance to settle. There are some lockticians that recommend waiting two to three months before shampooing baby locks to help speed up the locking process, but Sirca disagrees. Washing your hair less often will not have a significant effect on how quickly your hair locks and will only cause your hair to attract dirt, lint, and all sorts of other debris. Sirca also recommends going to an experienced locktician for your first shampoo. A professional locktician will show you how to wash your hair properly and how to deal with twists that come undone.

If, by chance, some of your locks start to unravel while washing your hair at home, don't panic. During this stage, your locks are highly susceptible to unraveling, especially if your hair is short (i.e. less than 3" long). This problem is also more common for individuals with soft, fine, or wavy textures than those with coarse or tightly coiled hair – but it can easily be fixed simply by re-twisting the affected areas. You can also prevent unraveling by covering your head with a nylon stocking *before* washing your hair. This practice can help keep your locks in place and prevent them from coming undone. For the most part, unraveling is somewhat unavoidable. At the end of the day, you must recognize this is just part of the locking process. Be patient and learn to deal with it.

During the three to four week period where you are not washing your hair, you can use witch hazel or an over the counter astringent like Sea Breeze to cleanse your scalp. Tea tree oil mixed with water can also be used to remove dirt and build-up from the scalp's surface. You may experience dryness and itchiness due to the alcohol content of these cleansers -- but applying Vitamin E or jojoba oil to the scalp will usually provide some relief.

"Using astringents to cleanse the scalp is still no substitute for actually washing your mane," warns Sirca. Since these cleansers can't eliminate the dust and odor trapped in your hair, at some point, you'll need to put down the Sea Breeze and cleanse your hair thoroughly to remove any dirt trapped in your hair and build-up on your scalp. *Remember:* clean hair is essential to growing healthy beautiful locks and your mane will thank you for it. If you suffer from a scalp condition, such as seborrhea, or lead an active lifestyle and need to wash your hair sooner, go right ahead. As a general rule, you should wash your hair anytime your scalp starts to feel dirty.

During the baby phase, your locks will start to swell and lose their tightly coiled shape. This is perfectly normal and just a part of the locking process. Your hair will also begin to matte together and form buds. Budding occurs when small pea-shaped knots begin to develop near the ends of your locks. Over time, these buds will become less apparent. Little balls of hair may also start to accumulate at the very tips of your hair. The formation of buds is completely natural and a sign that your locks are maturing. As far as the little balls are concerned, most lock wearers simply pull them off, so feel free to do the same.

This stage can be extremely difficult since your hair will lose its neat appearance and begin to look frizzy. Just avoid the temptation to pat your hair down, re-twist your locks, or hide under a baseball hat. I know you may be used to wearing nice neat hairstyles – but believe me, this is a time when your hair really starts to come into its own. Remember, the key to transitioning successfully into locks is to go with the flow and try to have fun with your locks as they grow.

Teenage Locks

Like a parent, you'll take great pleasure in watching your locks mature from a baby into a teenager. Although the teen years may be filled with difficult moments, during this time, you'll grow to better understand your hair. Depending on your hair texture, the method used to start your locks, and your maintenance habits, this stage can last anywhere from nine months to over four years. You'll also start to notice that your locks have started to lengthen and thicken. While your locks have started to settle, they haven't completely matured yet.

The tween and teen years bring a whole new set of challenges for lock wearers. This stage can be a lot like puberty, in that people grow insecure and frustrated with their hair as it develops. While your baby locks were cute, shiny, and easy to deal with: your teenage locks will undergo a lot of changes that may seem challenging or even daunting at times and require you to modify your maintenance routine ever so slightly. Knowing this in advance should help you to cope with any problems that may come your way. Trust in the knowledge that this is all part of a wonderful, new process that will eventually culminate in the new, beautiful locks you long for.

Maintaining Teenage Locks

Teenage locks should be washed gently every three to four weeks -- or more frequently depending on your lifestyle. If you exercise often, cleanse your scalp once a week with witch hazel and wash your locks every one to two weeks to help remove any odor or residue left on the scalp from sweating. Once your hair begins to matte, you can shampoo your hair more vigorously. At the same time, keep in mind you'll still need to handle your locks gently and with care.

Since teenage locks have the tendency to crawl together after shampooing, you'll want to inspect your roots to make sure that individual locks are not intertwining with one another. If they are, don't worry. You can fix the problem easily by gently pulling them apart at the roots while the hair is still damp. You'll also want to avoid letting too much time pass in between grooming sessions. Otherwise, it can cause damage to your locks and the separation process (when delayed too long) can become painful and more tedious.

Mature Locks

When your locks finally achieve adulthood, you'll look back and feel a tremendous sense of accomplishment and pride; your babies have finally grown up and are ready to shine and meet the world. Depending on your hair texture, you can expect your locks to reach their full maturity nearly four years after beginning the process. Although your locks may have settled, it can actually take additional time for them to assume their final shape and texture. After all that you have been through, this is the point where you should pat yourself on the back and congratulate yourself for having the perseverance and discipline to make it this far.

Maintaining Mature Locks

By now, you've probably developed a routine for caring and grooming

112

for your locks. Unlike baby and teenage locks, mature ones are stronger and require less maintenance. But before you get carried away, mature locks are still delicate. Remember, although your locks may look strong, they still must be handed gently and with care.

At this stage, there are a few more tips to keep in mind. When shampooing your mane, your goal should be to cleanse your scalp and to remove any dirt and lint trapped inside of your locks. As your locks grow and mature, your final rinse also becomes extremely important. After washing your hair, you'll need to make sure that you have completely removed all excess water and all traces of shampoo and conditioner. Sirca suggests "squeezing your hair repeatedly until the water runs clean to prevent residue from your shampoo and conditioner from building up inside your locks." With proper rinsing, you can generally eliminate the buildup left by styling aids and also cut down on drying time.

Sirca also recommends washing your locks in the bathtub or sink as they mature, so that you can focus exclusively on your hair. When people wash their locks in the shower, they have the tendency to rush through the process since their focus is divided between washing their body and hair. Shampooing in a bathtub or sink will ensure that your attention is focused on just your hair. Remember, the key is to cleanse your locks thoroughly.

One of the main benefits of having mature locks is being able to wash your hair more vigorously and frequently. Some mature lock wearers wash their hair daily while others wait anywhere from two to three weeks in between shampoos. With mature locks, you also have more freedom and flexibility when it comes to styling options. Now that your locks are longer, you can wear them pinned up in a number of styles, braid them and make them curly, or set them on rods for a wavy look. At this point, your styling options are unlimited!

Another advantage is that you no longer have to re-twist your new growth as frequently as you did when you had baby or teenage locks. However, there are some exceptions. Lock wearers with softer textures may need to re-twist with the same regularity throughout their entire lock journey. But in general, the need for certain types of maintenance decreases dramatically once your locks have matured.

Are We There Yet?

Instead of stressing over your mane, try to relax and enjoy the beauty of watching your locks transform. Some lock wearers become so focused on getting from point A to point B that they fail to take the time to appreciate their locks at all their different stages. Keep in mind that patience and dedication are critical to growing healthy, beautiful locks that everyone admires. There may be times when you feel impatient, stressed, or bored with your locks. But, there's no need to worry. If you take the time to cherish each phase, the journey will be that much more enjoyable. Just remember, anything in life worth having is worth working for.

Here are a few extra tips for dealing with the various issues that may arise in the process of growing and wearing your locks:

Removing Excessive Build-Up

If your locks start to look dry and dull, you may be suffering from product build-up. As with any hairstyle, a high quality clarifying shampoo will typically solve this problem – and remove the residue left by regular shampoos, conditioners, waxes, gels and pomades. But it should only be used occasionally. You can also make your own homemade clarifying treatment using apple cider vinegar and water. For a basic recipe, check out Chapter 15 – In the Kitchen. But be careful, if used too frequently (more than once a month), clarifying treatments can leave the hair and scalp feeling dry and brittle. For best results and to minimize dryness, always use a good moisturizing shampoo and/or a deep conditioning treatment following any clarifying treatment.

Drying Your Locks

Remember to dry your locks thoroughly and as quickly as possible. As your locks mature, they become denser and begin to absorb more water, which greatly increases drying time. To cut down the drying time, Sirca recommends towel blotting your locks immediately after washing your hair and sitting under a hood or bonnet dryer until your locks are close to dry. Sleeping on wet locks is also a No-No! This practice can leave your hair smelling like mildew and cause your locks to flatten out and lose their cylinder shape. Trust me, linguine shaped locks are not cute!

Dealing with Frizzies

Learning to deal with frizzy hair is just a normal part of having locks. If your goal is to have neat, manicured locks, stray hairs can be easily incorporated back into their respective lock with the palm-rolling technique. Just be careful to avoid over-twisting. Twisting your locks too frequently will cause them to weaken over time. Believe it or not, some people's locks become weak to the point that they fall right off!

Trimming Your Locks

Although your locks don't need to be trimmed as frequently as your hair when it was worn natural or relaxed, you should still have your ends clipped every four to six months to keep your locks looking healthy. Sirca *115* recommends cutting ½-1" off the ends to keep them in good condition -- but she says this amount can vary depending on your hair texture and how well you care for and maintain your locks.

Coloring Your Locks

Coloring locks is an extremely difficult process, which is best left to a professional. You may think you're saving money by coloring your locks at home, but if you make a mistake it could prove more costly at day's end. Plus, if your locks are long, you may wind up purchasing several boxes of color and spending close to what you would pay to have the service done in a salon.

If applied incorrectly, coloring can also be extremely damaging. Permanent colors will generally cause the most damage and if you're trying to alter your hair color by three or more shades, you can even change the texture of you locks. Choosing a shade that is close to your natural color will minimize the likelihood that damage occurs. Sirca also recommends using a good moisturizing shampoo and a deep conditioner at least once a month to keep color treated locks soft and healthy.

Color can be applied before or after the lock foundation is set. The most important thing to remember is that color should only be applied to hair in its healthy state. If your hair is weak or damaged, you should not be applying a color. The chemical process will only weaken your locks further and can ultimately result in breakage. For more tips on coloring your locks, check out Chapter 10 – Color Me Natural.

Veronica's Product Picks

In the beginning, your locks may look cute and shiny. But as time goes on, they can start to look dry and dull. This is to be expected. Unfortunately, most people try to remedy this problem with increased product usage. You may not feel the immediate effects of excessive product usage -- but over time, styling aids can start to build-up and cause your locks to appear dull and lifeless. You can avoid this result by using light, natural oils. Also, be sure to keep in mind like so many other things in life, when it comes to product usage, less is more.

When choosing a shampoo, you'll want to look for a product that will cleanse your scalp without stripping your hair of its natural oils. Sirca has found that moisturizing shampoos work best for lock wearers with kinky hair textures. Biolage Ultra-Hydrating Shampoo by Matrix is one that she recommends highly. For a conditioner that will leave your locks soft and moisturized, Sirca lists Biolage Ultra-Hydrating Balm by Matrix as one of her favorites. As a general rule, Sirca advices lock wearers to steer clear of creamy deep conditioners that coat the hair shaft and can result in residue build up inside of your locks.

When it comes to maintaining locks, pomades and locking butters are extremely popular. Many products are made with beeswax, petroleum, and lanolin – which coat the hair and wind up trapped inside of your locks over time. In the short-run, these products will hold your hair together and prevent unraveling -- but they can also be extremely difficult to remove and may cause your locks to look ashen and unhealthy. Instead, look for products that are light and can be easily absorbed by the skin. *Here's a test:* If you rub a little on your hand and it leaves a thick and

116

greasy film, you should consider using another product. Likewise, if you need heat to melt the product, don't use it on your hair.

Natural oils and alcohol-free styling gel offer a great alternative to heavy pomades. Sirca likes using light oils, such as jojoba, coconut, and sunflower oil -- which are easily absorbed by the hair and give it a nice shine. Natural oils are also great for keeping your locks soft and conditioned. In general, you only need to apply a few drops of oil, about the size of a quarter, to your hair ever couple of days.

For the best of both worlds, try adding a small amount of oil to your styling gel when you twist your hair for great sheen and hold. Although these are Veronica's picks, you may find that you get better results with other products. Experimenting with different styling aids is the key to growing beautiful locks --but remember: *It's always better to keep your product usage to a minimum.*

Taking Down Your Locks

There are many reasons why people decide to end their locking journey. Maybe you just want a fresh look or to start a new set of locks? Whatever the reason may be, it is important to know that you do have options.

The most common method of removing locks is by cutting them off. But you can actually save months, and even years of hair growth, by picking apart each lock. The entire *"take down"* process can be lengthy (several weeks or months) -- but it's well worth the time and effort if you've managed to grow your locks long.

If you plan on cutting your locks off, let your hair grow for at least one to two months. During this time, avoid re-twisting or manipulating your new growth to help ensure that the roots are as loose as possible. Once you have 1" of new growth, you can cut your locks off at the point where the roots and the locks meet and be left with a style, resembling a TWA. If you don't remember what a TWA is, don't worry. Just flip to the handy glossary in the back of the book.

Many salons also offer take down services. However, they can be extremely expensive due to the tedious nature of the process. If you prefer to take down your locks yourself, more details can be found on the next page.

Although you can remove your locks at home, I'm not going to sugarcoat things for you. It takes time and a fair amount of patience to undo this style properly. Just remember to be gentle with your hair, so that you can save as much of it as possible. During this process, it is quite likely that you'll experience some hair loss and a lot of shedding. This is completely normal. Keep in mind that the hair that you would ordinarily shed has been trapped in your locks for the duration of your entire journey. Since this process can take days, weeks, or even months -- depending on the length and thickness of your locks -- you'll want to start in the center near the back of your head, so that the hair can be pulled into a ponytail if you don't finish in one session.

118 *Note: the take down method may not be an option if you have manicured locks. If you have frequently clipped away loose strands to make your locks appear neater, you may find that you have an uneven mane once you complete the take down -- and may end up having to do a significant cut anyway.*

Take Down Instructions

What You'll Need
Shampoo
Deep Conditioner
Knitting Needle/ End of Rattail Comb
Take Down Cream (e.g. Kera Care Humectress Cream Conditioner)

- After shampooing and conditioning your hair, give yourself a deep conditioning treatment to help soften your locks. Once your locks have dried completely, snip off at least ½ – 1" off the ends of each lock so that you have a good starting point. The ends of your hair have been locked the longest, so they are often the most difficult to work with.

- Soak the ends of your locks in Take Down Cream to help loosen the hairs.

- Starting at the ends, use your fingers to pull apart the lock and work your way up to the root. If you get stuck along the way, squeeze a little Take Down Cream onto the matted section and let the solution saturate the hair for one to two minutes. Insert the knitting needle into the lock and use it to loosen the hair. Once you get pass this difficult section, continue to use your fingers to unravel the hair. Do not pull, tug, or rip through your hair with the needle or the comb as this can be damaging.

- When you have unraveled a lock completely, add conditioner and water to the loose hair. You can twist or braid this section so that it blends in with the rest of your locks OR you can opt to wear a scarf or head wrap until you have finished completely.

- When taking down locks, remove one lock at a time and comb through the unlocked section of hair thoroughly before moving on to the next one. This is extremely important and will help prevent your hair from becoming matted and tangled.

- Repeat these steps until each lock comes undone.

- TAKE A TRIP TO YOUR LOCAL NATURAL HAIR SALON AND HAVE A CONSULTATION WITH A STYLIST, WHO WILL BE ABLE TO ASSESS THE HEALTH AND CONDITION OF YOUR HAIR.

- WAIT AT LEAST FOUR TO SIX WEEKS AFTER TAKING DOWN YOUR LOCKS BEFORE HAVING ANY CHEMICAL SERVICE. YOUR HAIR IS IN A WEAKENED STATE AND IS EXTREMELY FRAGILE.

Growing locks is truly an individual process. What works for one person may not necessarily work for you. Whereas Janelle may only need to twist her hair every three weeks to keep them looking neat, Lacey may need to twist her hair every seven to ten days, because her hair texture is wavy and frizzes up easily. Again, everyone's locks are different. In fact, even on the same head, no two locks are exactly alike. Just be patient and do what's best for you and your hair. Remember, the goal is to spend less time fussing and fretting over your hair. Try and relax and enjoy this new look; have fun with the new you!

General Tips

Patience is a Virtue. Patience is extremely important when it comes to locking. You may find yourself growing frustrated at times, but try to relax and enjoy the journey. As with any type of hair style, there will be good days and bad days. Once you reach your goals, you'll be blessed with beautiful locks that represent this amazing experience.

Just Say No to Over-twisting. Twisting your locks everyday may keep your style looking neat, but it weakens your locks considerably over time. Sirca advises lock wearers to keep twisting to a minimum and discourages re-twisting more than once every two to three weeks.

Go Residue Free. Always wash your locks with a residue free shampoo. Regular shampoos made with fragrances and lubricants leave deposits behind that eventually build-up inside of your locks and slow down the matting process.

Sleep with a Satin Bonnet. At night, sleep with a scarf or satin bonnet to minimize damage caused by friction and to prevent the lint and fibers on your pillowcase from becoming trapped inside your locks. A satin pillowcase can also help to preserve your hair's moisture balance and reduces breakage.

Keep Mildew at Bay. Always be sure to dry wet locks thoroughly to keep them from mildewing. Remember, as your locks mature, they have the tendency to hold more water, which increases drying time and the chance that your locks will start to smell a tad bit moldy. Sirca also reminds lock wearers to NEVER sleep on wet locks.

Frizz is Normal. Every lock wearer should be prepared to experience a certain amount of frizz. For people with looser curl patterns, frizzies maybe something that you always have to deal with. Don't fret, it's normal.

Locks are Unique. Everyone's locks are different. Even on a single head, no two locks are exactly alike. Learn to love your locks just as they are and avoid comparing your locks to other's.

Avoid Beeswax. Steer clear of products containing beeswax, lanolin, and petroleum. Instead, opt for light oils -- which can be absorbed easily by the hair and shampooed out without much effort.

Water. Natural hair loves water. Sirca suggests spritzing your hair with water daily to help keep your locks hydrated in between washings. *121* Giving yourself a hot oil treatment once a month will also help to restore moisture to your locks and keep them looking and feeling soft and healthy.

Healthy Diet, Healthy Locks. Your hair, just like your body, needs a balanced and nutritious diet to stay healthy. Eating properly, staying hydrated, and taking care of yourself is essential to growing healthy and beautiful locks.

Key Points to Remember

- Locking is a lengthy process, which requires a major commitment and a tremendous amount of patience.

- Have a consultation with a professional locktician before starting your locking journey.

- Choose a locking method that fits with your lifestyle and budget.

- Handle your locks the way you would a fine piece of silk.

- Keep your product usage to a minimum.

122

Lock'd Styles

Get Lock'd Up

Baby Locks

Start off on the right track with a fresh pair of baby locks started by a professional locktician.

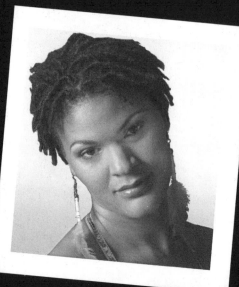

124

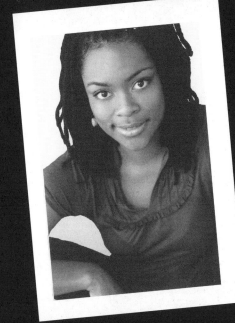

Teenage Locks

While teenage locks may be trying at times, this style is definitely worth the effort.

125

Mature Locks

Awww, mature locks, isn't wonderful to see how far your locks have come.

126

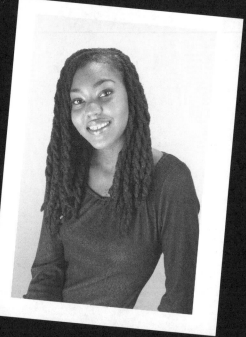

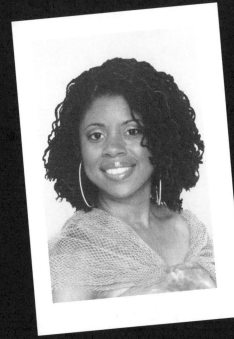

Sisterlocks

Clearly, there's no limit to style and versatility when it comes to having Sisterlocks.

127

Chapter 10
Color Me
Natural

When it comes to spicing up your look, coloring your hair is one of the quickest ways to give yourself an instant makeover. With just a few subtle highlights or complete coverage, you can instantly transform yourself into a sexy blonde, an alluring brunette, or an exotic ebony vixen. Color is also a powerful weapon in the battle against aging and can be a major confidence booster, even if the only thing that has changed is the hue of your natural hair. Whether you're looking to overhaul your look completely or simply enhance your natural shade, color has the amazing ability to take your style to the next level.

Experimenting with color can be fun and exciting. But as black women, we often face major challenges when it comes to dyeing our tresses. For starters, our hair tends to be dry and the color treatment process usually makes matters worse. The shape and texture of black hair can also make it difficult to achieve long-lasting color. Master colorist Lysa Ward, of the Georgetown Aveda Lifestyle Salon in Washington, D.C., has assured me, however, that with proper care and maintenance it is indeed possible to have healthy natural hair and color that stays fresh and vibrant in between salon visits. Thank goodness, right? Still, it is *129* important to remember that utmost care should be taken whenever you are considering color-treating your hair.

Selecting a Color

When selecting a hair color, be sure to choose shades that compliment your eye color and skin tone. In general, your skin tone is cool if your natural hair color is bluish-black, dark brown, medium ash, or golden blonde. If your natural hair color is red, golden brown, or deep brown with reddish highlights, then chances are you have warm tones. Most Latinas, Asians, and African-Americans fall into this category. One of the easiest ways to tell if your skin tone is cool or warm is by looking at the veins in your arm. If the veins have a bluish tint, then your skin tone is probably cool. If they are slightly greenish, then your skin tone is most likely warm.

Black women with cool tones tend to look best in ash shades, such as espresso, garnet, plum, and Bordeaux. If your skin tone is warm, go for chocolate, honey blonde, chestnut, or auburn hues. For a natural look, select a shade that is slightly lighter or darker than your normal hair color. The closer you stay to your original, natural color, the less your roots will show as they grow out. Naturals who opt for burgundy or chocolate shades can usually go anywhere from six to ten weeks without having their roots retouched. If you plan on going the honey blonde route, expect your roots to start showing in as little as three to four weeks. Plus, if funds are low and you are on a tight budget, you may want to opt for highlights instead.

Your best bet is to speak with a colorist, who can offer his or her professional opinion based on your skin tone and tolerance for upkeep. (So if you don't have one, get one! Don't know a good colorist? Ask your friends who colors their hair. There's nothing like a personal reference!) Ward strongly recommends discussing your color preferences with your stylist using photographs, color charts, and magazines to make sure that you are both on the same page. "What looks like auburn to you may look like honey blonde to your stylist," she says. Clear communication with your colorist is critical in order to avoid mishaps and ensure that you will be satisfied with the end result. Before taking the plunge, try wearing a wig or logging onto www.clairol.com, where you can upload photos of yourself and 'try on' color to get a better sense of how different colors will look on you.

Know the Difference

When dealing with color, your choice of permanent or semi-permanent hair dye can have a significant impact on your hair's health and overall condition.

Permanent Hair Color

Most permanent hair colors contain peroxide and/or ammonia and work by coloring and lightening the hair in one step. This process is referred to as single process hair color and is used to dye the hair darker colors with deep tones, like hot chocolate, chestnut, or auburn. Dyeing your hair honey blonde or sandy brown, however, involves bleaching the hair strand and requires the use of a double process hair color. "A double process hair color should only be performed by a professional -- and should never be attempted at home," says Sheila Head of Head Designs in Oakland, CA.

Permanent hair color should be touched up every four to six weeks, depending on how quickly your hair grows. Just be sure to keep in mind that your color will require more upkeep and maintenance the farther you stray from your natural shade. Permanent hair products can't be washed out, so you should give careful consideration to your choice of color before dyeing your hair. Most professionals, however, are capable of removing a permanent color and restoring your hair to its natural shade. But this process can dramatically impact both your wallet as well as the condition of your hair.

Semi-Permanent Hair Color

Semi-permanent hair color can be used to darken, but not lighten the hair. These products contain no or fairly small amounts of peroxide and are much gentler on your hair than permanent hair dyes. Semi-permanent dyes are nice because they produce bold and luxurious colors, without the drying and fading effects of permanent treatments. They also give the hair *131* an intense dose of color and a healthy looking shine.

Semi-permanent color can last from four to eight weeks and will fade gradually with each shampoo. These products are suitable for home use -- but Ward advises at-home users to "read and follow the instructions on the box carefully." The color produced by the chemicals in the box is only one aspect of the whole coloring process. The texture, condition, and other qualities of hair all impact how your hair will react to the coloring process. These are elements that typical home consumers are not prepared to address. In the end, unless you are very experienced, it's best to let the experts handle this process. Remember, all that advertising and slick packaging is meant to give you the illusion that you can color your hair yourself -- but it is just that, an illusion. So, be warned! In this, as with many things, mistakes can be not only costly, but also dangerous. 'Nuff said.

Natural Alternatives

If you're concerned about the long-term effects of using commercial hair dyes, then you may consider trying henna. Henna is an all-natural alternative to synthetic hair dyes and can be purchased at your local Whole Foods Market or General Nutrition Center. When used on black or dark brown tresses, henna gives the hair a deep auburn or burgundy tint, which fades gradually after several shampoos. Results may vary, however, depending on the texture and color of your natural hair.

If your mane is more than 10% grey, it isn't recommended that you use henna, which may turn your hair bright orange. If you've recently used a commercial hair dye, rinse, or relaxer, make sure you do a strand test first to determine how henna reacts with any chemical residue left on the hair. Despite their all-natural content, Ward strongly advises against using hennas because "they can be highly unpredictable and leave the hair feeling coarse and brassy with frequent use." Remember, just because something is all natural doesn't mean that there are no adverse reactions or risks involved.

132 Aveda is also among a growing number of companies that have started to produce herbal rinses and hair dyes made entirely from vegetable bases and botanical ingredients. Aveda's Full Spectrum line comes in over seventy-four shades ranging from pure black to blonde and is 97% derived from plant-based ingredients. Ward explains that Aveda's Full Spectrum Color System offers the widest range of permanent and depository shades to chose from, plus blonding formulas that require no bleaching. This line provides some of the most true-to-life tones enhanced with conditioners, such as sunflower, castor, and jojoba oils to improve the shine, quality, and strength of your tresses without the potential drying and damaging effects normally associated with chemical services.

Aveda has also developed a range of temporary color enhancing products made from mostly natural sources to seal in the effects of color enhancing shampoos, while also conditioning and detangling your hair. Ward counts Aveda products among her favorites, "because unlike many commercial dyes, they are gentle on the hair and leave it soft, shiny, and well moisturized."

Colored hair extensions are also a great way to go if you're just looking to add a few highlights and want the flexibility to change your color at a later date. Plus, extensions won't leave your strands feeling dry and brittle. Damage, however, may result from wearing extensions too long or if the hair is applied and/or removed incorrectly.

Color that Lasts

One of the most frequent complaints from black women with color is premature fading. Since the cuticle of kinky hair never closes completely, the molecular level is left exposed and the result is both natural and chemically induced fading. With over fifteen years of experience, Ward has managed to overcome this obstacle and has helped her clients with curly manes to achieve color that is long lasting. Here are Ward's tips to help you get the most out of your color and prevent pre-mature fading:

- **Keep maintenance in mind.** Always choose a color that is easy to maintain and fits with your lifestyle. "It's never a good idea for a low-maintenance woman to get a high-maintenance color," Ward says. If you are on a budget or tight schedule, opt for natural shades or highlights, that require less maintenance. Many women make the mistake of waiting until their color has faded to try and enhance it -- but you can easily extend the life of your color by taking proper care of it beginning with day one.

- **Wait at least two days after shampooing to color your hair.** The buildup of natural oils will help your hair to absorb the color more readily.

- **Deep condition.** Give your hue a boost, by doing a deep conditioner several days before you color your mane. A deep conditioner makes it easier for your hair to absorb the color and will give you longer lasting results. Plus, a good, deep conditioner can help to reduce any damage that may occur during the coloring process.

- **Use color-protective products.** Refresh your color by using a shampoo made for color treated hair in between salon visits. Color treated shampoos are gentler on the hair and often contain semi-permanent pigments that help the hair to maintain its bottled brilliance. For color that endures, try Aveda's plant-infused Color Conserve Shampoo made with organic lavender, organic ylang-ylang, and babassu nut to prevent your color from fading while protecting your locks from environmental stresses.

- **Minimize your exposure to sun and chlorine.** Sun and chlorine can damage your color and also cause your hair to feel dry and brittle. For added protection against chlorine, wear a swimcap or apply a leave in conditioner to your hair before you hit the pool. To reverse the harsh effects of chlorine and other harsh pool chemicals, try Aveda's Hair Detoxifier Shampoo formulated with certified organic aloe—to help maintain the hair's natural moisture.

- **Avoid overusing heated styling appliances.** As colored hair is prone to dryness and breakage, it is important to limit your usage of blowdryers or flat irons, which can cause color to fade and lead to split ends. If you must use heated styling appliances, make sure that they are set on the coolest possible setting. A thermal protector like *Aveda's Anti-Humectant or Damage Control* should also be used when blow drying or curling your hair.

- **Keep your hair moisturized.** Natural hair that is conditioned and well moisturized tends to hold color longer and have more shine. To keep your hair feeling soft and supple, Ward suggests using thick and creamy water-based conditioners. Try Aveda's Damage Remedy made with blends of sandalwood and barley to smooth the hair cuticle and quinoa protein – to help strengthen and repair hair from the inside out.

- **Use a color refresher.** Ask your colorist for a color refresher (mixture of shampoo and semi permanent color) to keep the color vibrant between touch-ups.

- **Trim your Ends.** Keep your color looking rich and vibrant by getting your ends trimmed every two to three months. Even if you are natural, getting your ends trimmed is a must in order to protect against split ends and breakage.

- **Read the label.** "Avoid styling products containing alcohol, which strip the hair of moisture and leave your tresses looking dull and lifeless" says Ward. Instead, look for moisturizing water-based syling aids rich in natural oils and conditioners. Try Aveda's Universal Styling Cream and Humectant, which Ward says work great on locks and twists; both tame frizziness while keeping hair vibrant and healthy.

Rich and vibrant hair color can be the ultimate accessory and the key to looking and feeling fabulous. Just remember, regular care and maintenance are both critical to achieving color that remains true over time.

Color At Home

When working with natural hair, technique is extremely important. *135* Because of its shape, color tends to show up darker on natural hair. For this reason, color expert Thierry Baptiste sometimes has to mix three or four different colors just to get the right shade. With at home color kits, women don't have the same control. "I have seen women come into the salon with pink, green, and orange hair -- just because they wanted to save $30 instead of having their hair colored professionally."

Although mistakes can be corrected, "most hair color disasters are caused by women who try to fix their own mistakes." Fixing a bad dye job can be tricky - so don't try to correct the problem by yourself. This will only make matters worse and cause further damage to your hair. Your best bet is to make an appointment with a professional colorist, who specializes in color correction. If you need to dye your hair at home to save funds or cut down on salon visits, here are some of Thierry's pro tips to help you avoid a hair coloring fiasco:

- **Do a patch test.** Save yourself a trip to the emergency room and do an allergy patch test on your skin at least 48 hours before each color application. Mercedes of Baton Rouge, LA learned this valuable lesson the hard way after being rushed to the hospital a few hours after coloring her hair. She suffered a severe allergic reaction to her favorite brand of color when the manufacturer's formulation changed. *Point to remember:* Never underestimate the importance of doing a patch test, even if you are only working with semi-permanent or temporary products.

- **Do a strand test.** Always perform a strand test before coloring your hair. Even if you are using the same color each time you dye your hair, you should still do a strand test to make sure the chemicals do not react differently due to any residues left on your hair or contaminants in the bottle.

- **Leave it to the pros.** Black hair is extremely delicate and can be easily damaged by harsh chemicals. If you're looking to change your natural color by more than three shades, leave the job to a professional! To locate an Aveda Salon in your area, check out www.aveda.com.

- **Read and follow the instructions on the box carefully.** "Aveda may require you to leave the solution on for twenty minutes, Dark & Lovely could say twenty-five, and Clairol may recommend thirty," says Baptiste. Each brand of hair color uses a different formula and should only be left on the hair for the time specified on the enclosed instructions.

- **Get organized.** Make sure you have a towel, a comb, a shower cap, gloves, and anything else you may need close by. Also, keep an extra bottle of dye on hand just in case you run out in the middle of coloring your hair.

- **Never dye your eyebrows or eyelashes at home.** An allergic reaction to hair dye could cause swelling, inflammation, and infection in the eye area -- and may even result in blindness. If you wish to have this service performed, contact Aveda for a salon offering brow and a lash tinting in your area

136

- **Ask for help.** "Don't be afraid to ask your stylist for advice on shades, product recommendations, or application tips," says Baptiste. Remember, your stylist's top priority should be helping you to achieve a healthy mane.

- **Ready, set, go!!!** If your color requires mixing, shake well and apply the solution to the hair immediately and discard any unused portion following use. The formula begins processing as soon as the color is mixed, whether you have applied it to your hair or not.

- **Roots only.** When touching up your color, apply the solution only to your roots to prevent breakage and over-processing. This technique will give you balanced coverage and a more uniform color from root to ends.

Risks and Warnings

In recent years, there have been growing concerns about the safety of synthetic hair dye. A study conducted by researchers at the Keck School *137* of Medicine at the University of Southern California found that women who regularly colored their hair with permanent hair dyes were at a much greater risk for bladder cancer.[22] Although the study only highlights the risk associated with dark colored permanent dyes and occupational hazards, Dr. Andrew Weil, natural health care guru and author of the best selling book *The Natural Mind*, advises against any use of hair dyes whatsoever. Many experts agree with Dr. Weil and recommend that if you choose to color your hair that you do it as naturally and as infrequently as possible. Until the results prove conclusive, here are some precautions you can take to limit your exposure to chemicals during the coloring process:

- Consider using herbal rinses or vegetable based products designed to add a hint of color.

- Never leave the dye on your head any longer than necessary.

- Rinse your scalp thoroughly with water after use.

- Wear plastic gloves and a mask when applying hair dye in order to reduce your exposure.

- Always read and follow the directions on the box carefully.

- Never mix different hair dye products because of potentially harmful reactions.

- Avoid scratching the head or scalp prior to any chemical service, as this may lead to irritation or even infection.

- If you're pregnant, be sure to consult with your doctor before coloring your hair. Many Ob/Gyns advise their patients to refrain from coloring their hair during the first trimester, while some doctors discourage their patients from receiving chemical services for the entire duration of their pregnancy.

Key Points to Remember

- Choose shades that compliment your eye color and skin tone.
- Select a color that is easy to maintain and fits with your own lifestyle.
- Always do a skin test before using any color product.
- For long lasting color, keep your hair moisturized and well conditioned.
- For best results, see a professional.

139

Chapter 11
The Perfect Blow Out

Tyra Banks, Kimberly Elise, and Mo'Nique can usually be seen sporting a super sleek mane with tons of body. What's the secret to their gorgeous, pin-straight locks? Emmy Award Winning stylist Lawrence Davis of Beverly Hills, California credits the perfect blow out. For the longest time, we, as black women, had only two choices when it came to straightening our hair. We could either get a perm and be left with strands that felt dry and brittle -- or a press 'n curl, which gave our kinky tresses a stiff and greasy finish. Fortunately, times have changed and now a growing number of us are discovering the secret of straightening our hair with just a blow dryer and a flat iron.

Having done hair for over fifteen years, Davis has perfected this technique and has been kind enough to give me the inside scoop on how to achieve a smooth and shiny mane. Read on to discover Davis' pro tips for obtaining straight hair with tons of body, minus the breakage and damage.

Healthy Natural Hair

By now, we all know that relaxers weaken our hair. But with a blowout, the hair's natural elasticity isn't compromised as much. As a result, this technique allows women to transition from curly to straight hair without concerns of over-processing. So, ladies, imagine! With this little secret in your hair war chest, relaxers will quickly become a thing of the past!

Transitioning

A major benefit of transitioning with a blow out is not having to cut your relaxed ends off all at once. However, if your hair has been badly damaged by chemical straighteners or you start to notice breakage in a lot of areas, you may need to do *The Big Chop*. Davis advises transitioners who prefer to wear their hair straight to have their ends trimmed frequently. "The sooner you cut off your relaxed ends, the easier your hair will be to maintain." Your mane will also look a lot fuller and healthier.

Learning to deal with moisture can also be a challenge for those who are transitioning with straight hair. You may be used to working out at full intensity or getting caught in the rain. However, when growing out your perm, sweat and humidity can wreak major havoc on your hair. This is just the reality of having to deal with two textures until your mane is fully trained. Tying down your hair with a scarf while exercising or carrying an umbrella when the weather forecast calls for showers can provide some relief -- but being patient and taking the time to understand your tresses will go a long way too.

Product/Styling Tips

When it comes to the blow out, having the right tools can make a world of a difference. To keep your tresses looking good in between salon visits, Davis suggests investing in both a good blow dryer and a flat iron. Today, modern appliances are far gentler on your hair than those from years past. Ionic blow dryers and ceramic irons now make it possible to achieve straight hair with luxurious shine and tons of body without the damage. Davis loves the FHI Heat Nano Salon Pro 2000 Blow Dryer, which uses natural ions to restore moisture balance to your strands. This blowdryer is lightweight, powerful, and leaves the hair silky straight. It also dries the hair in 20% less time, which helps to cut down on heat damage and breakage.

Ceramic flat irons are also a favorite among stylists who work with clients sporting natural hair. These irons have a remarkably smooth surface, which takes hair straightening to the next level. Ceramic irons are also designed to distribute heat evenly, helping to lock in moisture and giving the hair that silky-smooth salon finish. Davis highly recommends the FHI Heat Ceramic Flat Iron because it leaves your strands silky straight, giving your mane tons of shine, without having to use too many products. This iron also gives the user an amazing amount of control without pulling, breaking, or snagging your strands.

Depending on your texture, it can take up to a year to perfect your routine. "But once your mane is trained, its just like having a perm, minus the breakage," explains Davis. Using the right products and keeping your hair moisturized are both key to achieving head-turning locks. If you choose to wear your natural hair straight, Davis recommends using a rich moisturizing shampoo like Avalon Hydrating Shampoo and a conditioner chock full of vitamins and essential ingredients like Avlon Humecto Conditioner. For deep conditioning, try Joico Moisture Recovery, which leaves the hair feeling soft and silky to the touch.

Davis also likes Bumble & Bumble Brilliantine -- which is terrific for daily moisturizing. This super light pomade will keep your hair conditioned and help to minimize split ends. Once completely natural, Davis advises his clients who wear their hair straight to get a trim every four to six weeks. Usually, he finds that he doesn't have to cut as much off the ends, since their natural hair is generally in much better shape than when it was relaxed.

The Perfect Blow Out

With practice, you should be able to achieve the super sleek look you desire. To get you started, Davis has given me step-by-step instructions on how to blow dry and flat iron natural hair using the proper technique. Your stylist should also be able to give you additional tips for straightening your hair -- as well as product and styling recommendations. *143*

What You'll Need

- Anti Frizz Straightening Serum

- Blow dryer

- Ceramic Flat Iron with adjustable heat setting

- Sectioning Clips

- Rat-tail Comb

- Wide-tooth Comb

STEP 1. Start off with clean damp hair. After shampooing and deep conditioning, gently towel blot/dry the hair to remove excess water. Remove any knots and tangles by running a large-tooth comb through your hair. Remember, you'll want to start at the ends and work your way gradually up, towards the roots

STEP 2. Coat the hair with a straightening serum, such as Beyond the Zone Straight Shot Smoothing Serum, to make blow-drying the hair straight easier and to lock in shine and moisture. Distribute the product evenly by applying the serum to your hands first and then working it through your hair from roots to ends with your fingers. *Special Tip:* Apply more serum or gel to the curliest parts of your hair.

STEP 3. After applying the smoothing serum, part your hair into four to six sections of equal thickness, using a wide-tooth comb. For maximum straightening potential and even drying, twist each section tightly and secure with a large jaw clip. This process will help the hair to retain moisture and prevent your tresses from air drying and becoming frizzy.

STEP 4. For a smooth and glossy finish, sit under a dryer for ten to fifteen minutes before using a nozzled blow dryer. "You'll get much better results if you blow-dry hair that's almost 80% dry," he explains. *Special Tip:* Use a dryer with a nozzle to eliminate frizz and to concentrates the airflow on specific sections. Without a nozzle, the blowdryer gives off too much heat, which can dry out the strands and lead to damage and/or breakage.

STEP 5. Use a round, natural-bristle brush and a blow dryer set on a warm setting to straighten each individual section. *Note:* the diameter of the brush should be proportional to the length of your hair. If you have long hair, use a larger brush. The inverse is true for shorter hair. Make sure each section is completely dry before moving on to the next. As you blow dry your hair, always keep the airflow directed downward from the roots towards the ends. This technique smoothes the hair cuticle and results in straighter hair. Mastering this skill may sound relatively easy -- but you'll need to elevate the blow dryer above your head. This task can be difficult for people with short arms and also somewhat tiring over extended periods of time. Davis finds that drying your hair while sitting and holding the blow dryer over the top of your head puts less pressure on your arms and also makes it a lot easier to direct the air flow downwards.

STEP 6. For a salon sleek finish, apply a dollop of Bumble & Bumble Shine Serum to your palms. Rub your hands together, then smooth them over your hair to keep your style frizz-free.

STEP 7. After your hair has dried completely, part each section into smaller sections using a rat-tail comb. Working with smaller sections will help you to apply the iron's heat evenly and straighten the hair faster. Many women wonder why they don't get salon results with a flat iron. Sometimes, the problem has to do with trying to straighten too much hair at once. If you're working with sections that are too large, the outside layers of hair get the most heat, while the hair in the center is not heated enough. When the heat isn't distributed evenly, some parts of your hair end up feeling hard and frizzy, while others become silky straight.

STEP 8. Be careful! Ceramic irons get hot extremely quickly -- so avoid using a high heat setting to minimize hair damage. Go over each section with the flat iron slowly -- but be sure to keep the iron moving at an even pace. Try to get the flat iron as close to the roots as possible, then pull the iron slowly toward the ends. If necessary, run the iron over the hair a second time for a super-sleek finish. Continue, piece by piece, until your hair is completely straight. *Special Tip:* If you've never used a flat iron before, practice using it while it's turned off to get a feel for the device and the technique.

STEP 9. Finish with a light styling spritz like Avlon Dual Action Spritz.

A blow out is one of the best ways to temporarily straighten your curls without chemicals -- but it can take time and patience to perfect your technique. Just like with any other style, the key is practice, practice, practice! This is what it takes to get salon results.

Protect Your Strands

It should come as no surprise that you'll need to take precautions to protect your hair from heat damage caused by the straightening process. At night, you should continue to wrap your hair with a silk scarf and sleep on a satin pillow to prevent breakage. Instead of flat ironing your hair everyday, try wearing Velcro rollers in the shower in the mornings to give your hair a lift. You should also be diligent about your hair conditioning routine. Use a light daily moisturizer to keep your ends protected and do a weekly deep conditioner to keep your strands soft and conditioned. Finally, always apply a thermal protector to your strands before using a blow dryer or flat iron to guard against heat damage.

Davis also cautions women to think twice when they see signs advertising a $15 blow out. If it sounds too good to be true, it usually is. Salons that offer this service for cheap often end up damaging your hair in the long run. "They tend to use too much heat and don't know how to comb the hair out properly," says Davis. This, in combination with low quality products, can often lead to breakage and damage. So when it comes to hair straightening, just remember the old saying *"You get what you pay for."*

If you like the straight look, but aren't prepared to kiss your curls goodbye, then you'll want to save your blow dryer and flat iron for special occasions. *Note:* if you straighten your hair too frequently, you can permanently alter your natural curl pattern -- which may prevent you from experimenting with natural styles that require texture and volume. Just remember the only way to fix this problem is by cutting your straight ends off and allowing your natural texture to grow out again.

Although I may personally prefer to don a wig or sew in a weave for special occasions, many women love the look and feel of wearing their natural hair straight. The good news is that both alternatives leave you with healthy tresses and minimize the breakage and damage caused by relaxers. This natural style is also a great option if you desire to grow your hair long or are just looking to get glammed up for a special occasion. Plus, with the wide range of styling products and straightening appliances on the market, it's now easier than ever to get the chic, shiny look you so desire. Moderation is key -- so just be sure to take it easy on your locks.

146

Key Points to Remember

- Steer clear of the $15 blow out.

- Get your ends trimmed frequently to make caring for your hair easier.

- Keep your mane moisturized and well-conditioned.

- Invest in a good blow dryer and flat iron to keep your locks looking good in between salon visits.

- Straightening your hair too frequently can permanently alter your natural curl pattern.

147

Chapter 12

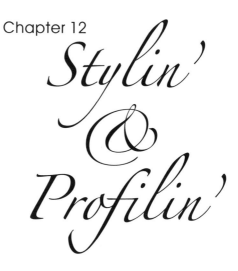

Stylin'
&
Profilin'

If you're tired of flipping through the pages of black magazines and seeing so-called natural styles created with fake hair and human extensions, there's no need to look any further. Most of the styles found on the following pages were created without extensions using only the model's natural hair. These styles are modern, professional, and chic – and best of all, they are easy to pull off. What's more, these ladies have no problem getting a date or holding down a job. And the great thing is that with minimal time and practice, you can easily master these 'dos at home. That means you can put that extra $50 in your pocket and spend it on a new pair of shoes or a nice dinner -- or however else you see fit. For step-by-step instructions on how to recreate these styles, check out my website **www.thankgodimnatural.com**.

Now that you're ready to take the plunge, turn the page and find many sources of inspiration for healthy, fabulous, and natural hair.

* * * *

149

Caesar

Kiss bad hair days goodbye with this short sexy do. The style is bold and daring -- but also shows off your soft, feminine side. Keep things interesting by experimenting with your hair color, makeup, and jewelry.

150

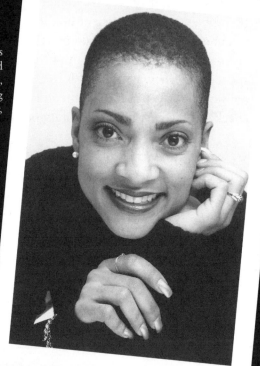

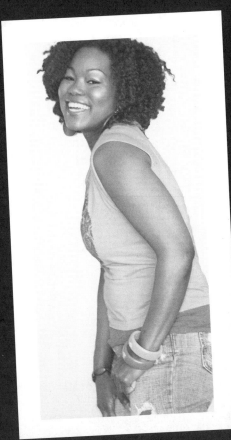

Twist Out

Take your mane for a fabulous turn with this beautiful twist out. This free flowing style gives the wearer a relaxed and casual look. This do also looks great on kinky textures and makes a major mane statement.

151

Bantu Knots

This style is for you ladies with plenty of confidence. You can work this look on the weekend and take the knots down on Monday for a beautiful twist out. Whether you're coming or going, this do stays fresh and funky.

152

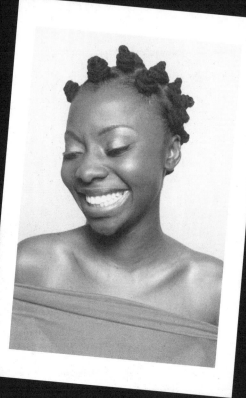

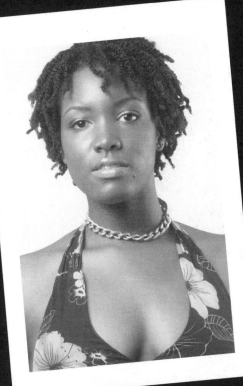

Kinky Twists

Keep your hair looking tight everyday with
these magnificent, kinky twists. Pull them
back, pin them up, or just wear them loose.
This protective style is also great if you are
looking to give your hair a break from the
daily rigors of brushing and combing.

153

Afro Puff

Looking for a drama free look? Well your search is over! This drawstring afro puff ponytail offers style and convenience and will take you from nine to five with very little effort.

154

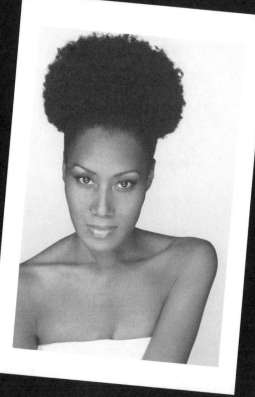

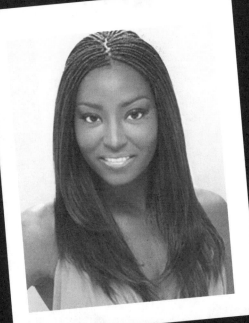

Microbraids

This classic, all-time favorite is perfect for those ladies who are on the go or who love to get their exercise on. This protective style will also give your hair a break from daily styling and manipulation. For a different look, try using wet and wavy hair or working with highlighted extensions.

Weave

Get the look of straight hair -- minus the damage caused by heat styling -- with a sew-in weave. This sassy 'do gives the wearer tremendous flexibility and can be styled in a number of different ways. But don't be fooled. A weave requires work! If you don't have the time or the money to keep your extensions looking tight, opt for a style with lower maintenance. Also, check out Chapter 7 for more tips on how to keep your extensions looking good.

156

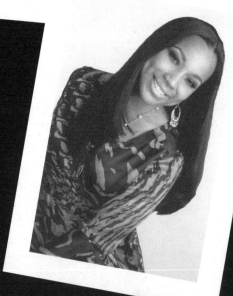

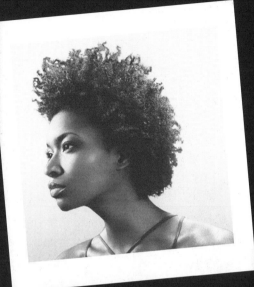

Chunky Fro

When Jill Scott hit the scene wearing this style, she brought a modern flair to this old throwback. Since this look is all about funk and soul, you can rock this free flowing 'do from sun up to sundown -- without ever worrying about a single hair being out of place.

157

Locks

What more is there to say about locks? This beautiful natural style requires commitment -- but it's definitely worth it, especially once your mane reaches its full potential

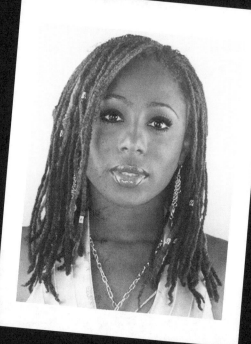

158

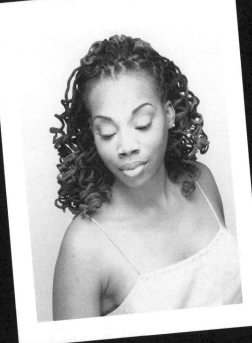

Crinkly Locks

These sexy tendrils bring new meaning to the word subtle beauty. Big flowing waves give this model a soft, romantic look and scores major points in the elegance department.

159

Lock Updo

Keep it simple and elegant with a beautiful lock pin up. Undeniably playful and sexy, this romantic updo is the perfect look for just about any special occasion.

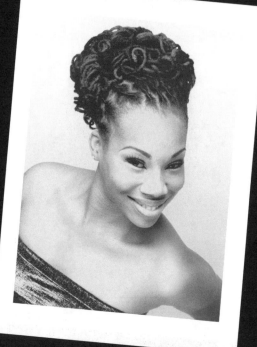

160

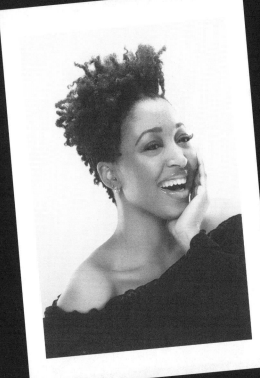

Faux Hawk

Show off your daring side with this stylish faux hawk. This bold and edgy look is FIERCE and will definitely make you stand out in the crowd.

Natural Ponytail

Feeling fun and flirty? Take it there with this high natural ponytail. This carefree do is the official definition of natural chic.

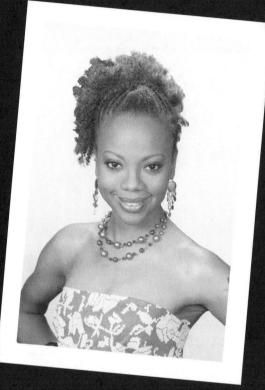

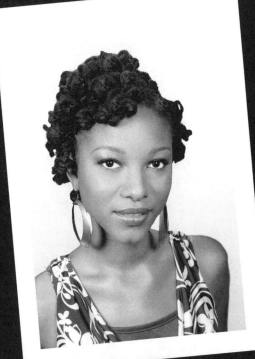

Coiled Locks

Pinned-up coils gives this maven touchable
tendrils for a style that always measure up.

163

Blow Out

If you're looking for a smooth and sleek style, you can't go wrong with a press n' curl. You'll score plenty of compliments with this sophisticated 'do and have everyone asking for your stylist's phone number.

164

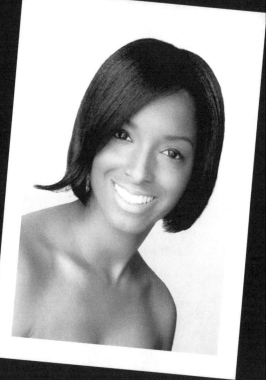

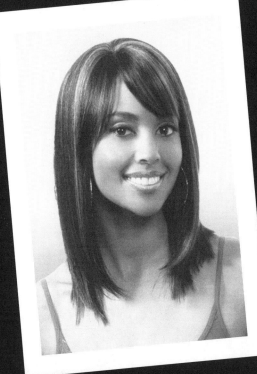

Wigs

Give your hair a break with a nice stylish wig. Go for a short, flirty bob or glam it up with a shoulder-sweeping style. For just $24.99, you can transform your tresses from kinky to straight with no heat and very little effort.

165

Lock Ponytail

This lockponytail shows there is no shortage of options when it comes to this style. This low maintenance do has just enough flair and sophistication to give the wearer a nice polished look that's perfect for just about any occasion.

166

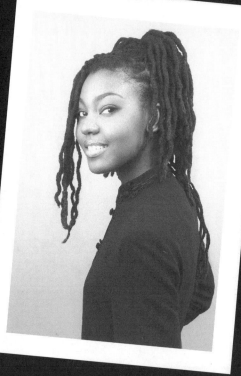

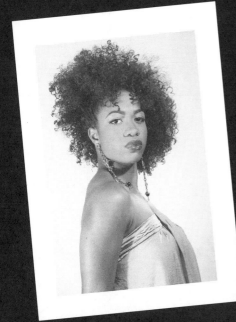

Flexi Rod Set

For a little more pizzazz, play up your sassy side with a flexi rod set. This mane, full of perky ringlets, is soft and touchable and gives your hair a major style boost. Rod sets are also gentler on the hair than styles that require the use of a curling iron and the curls are long lasting. For another look altogether, try experimenting with different size rods or changing the amount of hair you place on each rod.

167

Chapter 13
Product Picks

Walk through the aisles of any beauty supply store and you'll find hundreds of products, all of which promise to improve the texture, quality, and manageability of *black hair*. But don't be fooled by the brown shampoo bottle or the red, black, and green label. There simply is no one-size-fits all solution for grooming and caring for kinky tresses. Your girlfriend might use a pomade that gives her curls tons of body and shine -- but the same product may leave your hair feeling dry and crunchy.

When it comes to choosing the right products, knowing whether your hair is dry, oily, normal, or combination can make all the difference and save you lots of time and money spent on brands and routines that don't work. Although there are many systems for classifying hair, your strands generally fall into one of four main categories. With so many options to choose from, it can be overwhelming figuring out which products to try. To make life easier, I've compiled a list of the best styling aids based on your hair's specific characteristics.

Dry Hair

Although there are always exceptions, the general rule is the smaller the curl, the drier the hair. Dry hair doesn't have much of a shine -- but with the right products, it can give off a nice sheen. Dry hair also tends to be fragile and breaks very easily. When it comes to styling and caring for dry hair, the following products will keep your locks moisturized and well-conditioned:

Shampoo - For dry hair, try Nature's Gate Chamomile & Lemon Verbena Moisturizing Shampoo for Dry, Damaged Hair. This extra-gentle moisturizing shampoo is infused with chamomile and lemon verdbena, which strengthens, softens, and enhances your hair's natural shine. *Product Tip:* Limit your use of volumizing and clarifying shampoos, which tend to strip the hair of its natural oils.

Conditioner - For extra moisture and major shine, try Uans Crema Conditioner. This specially formulated conditioner restores softness, silkiness, and manageability to dry, damaged, and chemically treated hair.

Deep Conditioner - For extra-dry hair, use Aveda's Damage Remedy Intensive Restructuring Treatment once a week. This ultra rich, deep conditioner is infused with rich shea butter and avocado cream oil, which helps restore moisture and elasticity to your natural curls.

Pomade /Moisturizer - Dry hair needs moisture -- not grease or heavy pomades that weigh the hair down and cause product build-up. For a daily moisturizer that will condition your curls and give you a smooth finish, Kenyon Hall, owner of Time Hair Gallery in Chicago, recommends Jane Carter's Solution Nourish & Shine. Made from pure shea butter and mango butter, this delectable treatment will leave your hair smelling good, without too much product build-up or residue.

Oily Hair

If you spend thirty minutes every morning styling your hair and by noon it looks greasy and lifeless, join the club. You're just one of millions of people born with oily hair. Oily hair is caused by overactive sebaceous glands, which produce the natural oils that keep our hair soft and supple. These natural oils also offer added protection against breakage and split ends. When natural oils build-up on the scalp, they attract dust and dirt -- which cause the hair to appear dull and lifeless. This also explains why women with oily hair need to wash their hair more frequently. Nedjetti of Hair by Nedjetti in Bloomfield, NJ recommends the following products for use on oily hair:

Shampoo - If oily hair is a problem, try a deep cleansing shampoo like Soy Cream Shampoo by Blended Beauty. You'll be amazed at how this shampoo removes build-up from the scalp without stripping your strands of their much-needed natural oils. Adding one teaspoon of lemon juice to your regular shampoo will provide similar results. *Product tip:* Avoid conditioning or moisturizing shampoos, which weigh hair down and may cause it to look and feel greasy. Also, steer clear of creamy shampoos and go straight for the clear ones, which tend to contain stronger cleansing agents. *Maintenance tip:* For extra oily hair, leave the shampoo on your scalp for three to five minutes in order to remove any excess oil or residue.

Conditioner - When it comes to conditioners, you'll want to choose a light product that won't leave your hair flat and limp. For oily hair, try Quenching Conditioner by Blended Beauty. This intense, luxurious hair conditioner is extra moisturizing and full of nutrients to keep hair healthy and growing. Formulated with chamomile and rosemary extract, this hydrating conditioner restores moisture balance and leaves the hair soft and silky to the touch. *Style tip:* Be sure to apply the conditioner only to your ends and not your roots.

Deep Conditioner - Since your scalp is already doing its job of keeping your strands well moisturized, you're probably better off skipping the deep conditioner.

Pomade/Moisturizer - Oily hair doesn't require much in the way of product. Stick to light oils and/or pomades for styling and avoid products containing silicone, petroleum, or lanolin. These products are usually heavy and can cause your scalp to produce more oil. For a light, non-greasy moisturizer, try Curly Frizz Pudding by Blended Beauty.

171

Normal Hair

Normal hair is hair that is neither oily nor dry. Women with this hair type can usually go several days without washing their hair, because there is no excess build-up on the scalp. This hair type also has a natural shine. The key to caring for normal hair is choosing styling aids that will maintain your hair's natural moisture balance. The following products are formulated specifically for normal tresses and will leave you with fabulous healthy hair.

Shampoo - Improve and maintain your hair's natural moisture balance with Aveda's Rosemary Mint Shampoo. Formulated with peppermint to awaken your senses and rosemary to protect your locks from environmental damage, this mild shampoo will leave the hair feeling soft and silky, while enhancing body and shine.

Conditioner - For the normal hair type, try Aveda's Rosemary Mint Conditioner. This conditioner is enriched with natural ingredients, which revitalize the scalp and leave the hair feeling soft with a glossy shine.

Deep Conditioner - Biolage Ultra-Hydrating Balm by Matrix is an intense treatment mask that strengthens, protects, and nourishes. This hydrating concoction is made with lemongrass and wheat germ – both of which help to replenish moisture and restore hair to good health.

Moisturizer - When dealing with normal hair, try Ashea's Shea Butter Pomade. This lightweight moisturizer is made with pure shea butter and a blend of herbal ingredients to impart shine and softness to your locks.

Combination Hair

Many women have what is called combination hair. This type of hair is oily at the scalp and dry at the ends. Combination hair is fairly common in people with dandruff, because the dry flakes on the scalp absorb the hair's natural oils. Caring for this hair type, while challenging, need not be a nightmare. With the right products and proper maintenance, Natasha Jackson of Na'Klectic Hair Gallery in Baltimore, MD, says "you can keep combination hair looking healthy and fabulous." Here are some of Natasha's faves for combination hair. Give them a try and see if you like them for yourself.

Shampoo - If you have combination hair, avoid using shampoos made for oily hair. These products contain deep-cleansing agents, which may cause further damage to already dry ends. Instead, opt for shampoos formulated for normal hair and concentrate on applying the product to your ends. A good shampoo for combination hair is Jason Natural's Vitamin E with A & C Shampoo. It's chocked full of natural ingredients that will clean and clarify your oily scalp.

Conditioner - Jason Natural's Vitamin E with A & C Conditioner is lightweight and great for combination hair. This oil free conditioner restores moisture balance and leaves the hair soft and shiny, but not greasy.

Deep Conditioner - Give your combination locks some extra TLC with a deep conditioner once a week. Try using Miss Jessie's Rapid Recovery and focus on applying the product to the dry parts of your hair. This rich, hydrating conditioner will restore luster and shine to dry ends without leaving your scalp feeling oily or greasy.

Pomade /Moisturizer - Stick to light oils or pomades containing natural ingredients. Nature's Blessings Virgin Olive Oil is a great lightweight moisturizer for combination hair -- with a fresh citrus scent to keep your hair smelling wonderful all day long.

Are Salon Products Really Better?

In general, salon products tend to be of higher quality than the products sold at your local beauty supply or drugstore. This is true in most cases -- but not all. "Salon products typically contain gentler cleansing agents and higher quality protein based or moisturizing conditioners that lock in moisture," says Lysa Ward of Aveda Georgetown Spa and Lifestyle Salon in Washington, D.C.. These quality ingredients also contribute to the higher cost of salon brands. As with any product, however, there will be expensive brands that do nothing for your hair and cheaper ones that will give you amazing results. Your best bet is to experiment with different products until you find the right combination that works for your hair.

* * * *

Knowing whether your hair is dry, oily, normal or combination will help you to choose products that will keep your locks looking healthy, beautiful and natural. Buying products specially formulated for your hair will also save you time and money – and avoid costly hair care mistakes. While using the products recommended in this chapter will certainly improve the condition of most people's hair, always be sure to conduct a strand test first in order to determine the effect the products will have on your hair.

Key Points to Remember

- Knowing your hair type can save you time and money on brands and routines that do not work.

- Invest in quality products made specifically for your hair type.

- Less is always more.

Disclaimer: Degrees of success in hair styling varies greatly depending on your hair texture, type, and condition. Thank God I'm Natural assumes no liability or responsibility for any damages or injuries that may result from the products described herein. Please carefully read all information provided on or in the product packaging and labels to determine whether you have any allergies or sensitiveness before use. Thank God I'm Natural also advises readers to consult their own physician with respect to the safety and efficacy of any product.

174

175

Chapter 14

"Natural"? Beware!

In this day and age, where the word *"natural"* is synonymous with *"healthy"*, companies are all too eager to jump on the organic bandwagon to satisfy our appetites for so-called wholesome living. In recent years, the market has become saturated with shampoos, lotions, and moisturizers that claim to be *"natural"*, but whose ingredients are barely distinguishable from their artificial counterparts. Believe me, these natural imposters are everywhere, including your local health food co-op.

But what, if anything, can you do to protect yourself? While it may seem daunting, you can arm yourself with knowledge and become a smart shopper – which will help you make the right decisions as a consumer. So, let's start with the basics and consider what *"Natural"* really means when you see it printed on various cosmetic products.

Why Natural?

What we put on our bodies is just as important as what we put in our bodies. Our skin is our largest organ and has the remarkable ability to absorb substances into the bloodstream. As you might guess, this can be both a good and bad thing; good, because we can deliver vital nutrients and sustenance to our bodies easily via our skin; bad, because many lotions, moisturizers, and shampoos contain harmful ingredients that should never be ingested into the body -- orally or otherwise.

Of the tens of thousands of chemicals that have been developed in the last half-century, very few have been assessed for safety for their long-term effects on human health and the environment.[23] Surely then, it's no great coincidence that the incidence of illnesses such as eczema and allergies have increased over the same time period and that cancer rates have now reached epidemic proportions. While it's not possible to avoid all contact with harmful substances, we can certainly minimize our interaction by switching to products that are truly all natural by always remaining vigilant and focused on the ingredients list.

Reading the Label

The biggest mistake women (and many men too!) make when shopping for a shampoo or a conditioner is looking for pretty labels. Let me tell you, chic packaging is nothing more than eye candy. Reading labels is the **ONLY** sure-fire way to gather information about the ingredients contained in your hair care products so you can make smart purchasing decisions. This information can also be useful in helping you determine which styling aids to purchase and to understand why certain products are heavy, greasy, or drying to your hair. Companies may (sometimes intentionally) choose to make product packaging confusing. But we as consumers must do our homework. So take a deep breath, get out your magnifying glass, and let's tackle the ingredient list!

In cosmetics, ingredients are listed in descending order by weight. Ingredients present in the largest concentration are always listed first -- while those present in smaller amounts are listed last. You'll typically see water (aqua) listed as the first ingredient in most products and colors and fragrances listed towards the end of the label. Any ingredient present in a concentration of 1% or less may be listed in any order, so long as it is listed after all the ingredients present in a concentration greater than 1%. Note, there is no requirement that manufacturers disclose where the 1% cutoff begins on the label. Finally, when you see the words *"and other ingredients"*, it means the FDA has granted a manufacturer trade secret status for a particular ingredient and they are not required to disclose it at all.

Often, you'll come across words on an ingredient list that appear to be in a different language. In this case, the manufacturer is complying with the International Nomenclature of Cosmetic Ingredients (INCI), a multinational system based on Latin for naming cosmetic ingredients. The INCI forms the basis of the ICI Dictionary and Handbook, which presents, in detail, the bulk of INCI names juxtaposed with their technical/trade names to allow for their easy identification. Below is a chart of just some of the names in the INCI system for ingredients commonly found in hair products. However, don't be alarmed immediately if you see ingredients listed in this format. Many of them are still perfectly healthy – even if they are described in this INCI system. What's essential is understanding what the various ingredients actually mean to you, the consumer.

INCI Naming System

	INCI Nomenclature (proper INCI name)
Almond Butter	Hydrogenated Almond Oil
Almond Oil	Prunus Amygdalus Dulcis (Sweet Almond) Oil
Avocado Oil	Persea Gratissima (Avocado) Oil
Babassu Oil	Orbignya Oleifera (Babassu) Seed Oil
Baking Soda	Sodium Bicarbonate
Beeswax (block or pastille)	Beeswax
Bentonite Clay	Bentonite
Benzaldehyde FCC	Benzaldehyde or Fragrance or Flavor
Calendula Extract	Calendula Officinalis OR Calendula Officinalis Flower Extract
Carrot Seed Oil	Daucus Carota Sativa (Carrot) Seed Oil
Chamomile Extract	Chamomilla Recutita (Matricaria) Flower Extract
Clay, Bentonite	Bentonite
Clay, China	Kaolin
Coconut Oil	Cocos Nucifera (Coconut) Oil
Cornstarch	Zea Mays (Corn) Starch
Emu Oil	Emu Oil
Hemp Seed Oil	Cannabis Sativa (Hemp) Seed Oil
Jasmine Oil	Jasminum Officinale (Jasmine) Extract
Jojoba Oil	Simmondsia Chinensis (Jojoba) Seed Oil
Lavender Oil	Lavandula Angustifolia (Lavender) Oil
Lemon Oil	Citrus Medica Limonum (Lemon) Peel Oil
Mango Butter	Mangifera Indica (Mango) Seed Butter
Nettle Extract	Urtica Dioica (Nettle) Extract
Oat Bran	Avena Sativa (Oat) Bran
Olive Oil	Olea Europaea (Olive) Oil
Orange Oil	Citrus Aurantium Amara (Bitter Orange) Oil

Palm Butter	Hydrogenated Palm Oil
Peppermint Oil	Mentha Piperita (Peppermint) Oil
Pink Graefruit Peel Oil	Citrus Paradisi (Grapefruit) Peel Oil
Rose Geranium Oil	Pelargonium Graveolens Oil
Rosehip Oil	Rosa Canina Fruit Oil
Seaweed Extract	Fucus Vesiculosis Extract
Sesame Seed Oil	Sesamum Indicum (Sesame) Seed Oil
Shea Butter, Natural	Butyrospermum Parkii (Shea Butter) Fruit
Spearmint Oil	Mentha Viridis (Spearmint) Leaf Oil
Sugar	Sucrose
Sunflower Oil	Helianthus Annuus (Sunflower) Seed Oil
TEA	Triethanolamine
Tea Tree Oil	Melaleuca Alternifolia (Tea Tree) Oil
Vegetable Glycerine	Glyrcerin
Vitamin A	Retinol
Vitamin E	Tocopherol
Water	Water OR Aqua OR Onsen-Sui
Wheat Germ Oil	Triticum Vulgare (Wheat) Germ Oil
Ylang Ylang Oil	Cananga Odorate Flower Oil
Yucaa Herbal Extra	Yucca Schidigera Extract

The Bad Guys: Ingredients to Avoid

Knowing which ingredients to avoid is just as important as figuring out what ingredients to look for. If you have a strong preference for using natural products, here are ten ingredients to steer clear of the next time you go shopping for shampoo:

1. **Sodium Lauryl/Laureth Sulfate (SLS)** — is a detergent used in most shampoos, shaving creams, and bubble baths for its cleansing and foaming properties. Like most harsh detergents found in your shampoo, SLS strips the hair of its natural oils -- often leaving it dry and brittle. SLS may also cause eye irritation, scalp scurf similar to dandruff, skin rashes,

and other allergic reactions. Be on the lookout for the words "comes from coconut." SLS is frequently present in pseudo-natural products under this description. Although there are many websites claiming SLS is a carcinogen, the American Cancer Society has taken the position that SLS and Sodium Laureth Sulfate (SLES) do not cause cancer.

2. **Diethanolamine (DEA), Triethanolamine (TEA)** — These ingredients are used to stabalize the pH of most personal care products. Depending on the individual, DEA and TEA may cause allergic reactions and eye irritation, as well as dry hair and skin. Neither DEA nor TEA is carcinogenic. However, if either of these compounds interact with nitrites - often present as contaminants in personal care products, a chemical reaction may result, which can lead to the creation of cancer-causing nitrosamines. In recent years, many companies that sell "natural products" have been caught using DEA and TEA in their cosmetic preparations.

3. **Parabens (Methyl, Propyl, Butyl and Ethyl)** — Parabens are the most commonly used preservative in shampoos, conditioners, and other styling products. The antimicrobial properties of these chemicals help to extend the shelf life of most cosmetics and personal care products by two to three years. Parabens have long been considered safe -- but a few recent studies have suggested that these chemicals may actually lead to breast cancer. The validity of these studies have been challenged due to the lack of experimental evidence, but such alarming claims continue to be the subject of further investigation.

4. **Diazolidinyl Urea, Imidazolidinyl Urea** — After parabens, ureas are the most commonly used preservative in cosmetics and personal care products. Under certain circumstances, exposure to ureas may cause contact dermatitis.

5. **Lanolin, Petroleum and Mineral Oil** — These cheap ingredients are widely used in greases and pomades formulated for black hair and offer no real moisturizing benefits. In fact, these ingredients often weigh the hair down and prevent the natural oils produced by the scalp from being absorbed by the hair shaft. For a natural alternative, try jojoba, coconut, or sweet almond oils for their conditioning properties.

6. **Propylene Glycol** — This humectant is commonly found in shampoos, lotions, after-shave, deodorants, mouthwashes, and toothpastes to give a product "glide" or "slip." This chemical is also an active ingredient in anti-freeze, airplane de-icer and brake and hydraulic fluid. Recent findings indicate that propylene glycol may cause allergic reactions, dermatitis, dry skin, hives, and eczema. Because it is easily absorbed by the skin, the Environmental Protection Agency has issued a mandate requiring workers to wear protective gloves, clothing, and goggles when handling this toxic substance.[24] Material Safety Data Sheets also warn against skin contact with this agent, because it has been shown to cause brain, liver, and kidney abnormalities. Beware of PEG (polyethylene glycol) or PPG (polypropylene glycol)—they are related synthetics.

7. **Synthetic Colors** — Artificial colors are used widely in hair care products for aesthetic purposes. These ingredients frequently appear as FD&C or D&C followed by a color and a number (e.g. FD&C Red No. 6 / D&C Green No. 6). Color pigments may cause skin sensitivity and irritation. The safety of these ingredients is also questionable -- because they are derived primarily from coal tar, a known carcinogen.

8. **Synthetic Fragrances** — Synthetic fragrances are present in most shampoos, conditioners, and styling pomades. The word "fragrance" can indicate the presence of up to 4,000 separate ingredients, many of which are synthetic.[25] In some individuals, these compounds can induce headaches, dizziness, rash, skin discoloration, violent coughing, vomiting, and skin irritation. For a safe alternative, try purchasing unscented products from your local Whole Foods Supermarket and adding your own fragrance using all-natural essential oils.

9. **Formaldehyde** — This cheap preservative is used in hair care products containing water to prevent the growth of bacteria. Formaldehyde is a suspected carcinogen and may cause skin reactions, trigger heart palpitations, or lead to joint pain, allergies, headaches, chest pains, ear infections, and dizziness. Despite its possible harmful side effects, cosmetic manufacturers are free to use formaldehyde in your shampoos, conditioners and lotions without listing it as an ingredient.

10. **Coal Tar** — Many shampoos designed to treat dandruff contain

coal tar -- although it's frequently absent from the product's list of ingredients. Protect yourself and be on the look out for this compound, which is disguised in many forms (e.g. "Stantar", "Clinitar", "Medi-Tar" and "Polytar"). While the FDA acknowledges that coal tar is a carcinogen under certain conditions, it has taken the position that it still safe for use as an active ingredient in most over-the-counter dandruff shampoos. Not surprisingly, most shampoo manufacturers are in agreement and continue to use it. Still, in addition to being a cancer hazard, coal tar has been found to cause allergic reactions, asthma attacks, headaches, nausea, fatigue, nervousness, and lack of concentration.

Manufacturers often make the argument that these and other synthetic ingredients pose no real, serious threat to our health and safety since they are present in personal care products in such small amounts. Even if this were true, it is hard to believe that these chemicals will not have some long-term effect on our bodies after we've been exposed to them day after day, year after year. If you frequently suffer from any of the symptoms described above, you may want to check the list of ingredients on your hair and skin care products. If you have children or sensitive *183* skin, you should also be mindful that chemical additives and synthetic ingredients can sometimes cause allergic reactions even in small doses. Your best bet for protecting yourself and your family is to avoid products containing high concentrations of synthetic ingredients and to look for natural alternatives whenever possible.

The Good Guys: Ingredients to Look For

Not all products are bad for your hair or your health. If you're not sure what to look for in your shampoo and conditioner, here is a list of ten natural ingredients that are great for black hair. Just remember, you'll want to purchase products, where these appear towards the beginning of the list of ingredients. Please note that some of these items are also available for individual purchase and can be added to your hair products separately for their beneficial properties.

1. **Shea Butter** — Shea butter is a natural fat extracted from the fruit of the Karite tree, which grows in Western Africa. Because of its

conditioning properties, this natural moisturizer is used in hair dressings and pomades to restore moisture to dry brittle hair, prevent breakage and split ends, and promote healthy hair growth.

2. **Aloe** — This natural moisturizer is frequently used in shampoos and pomades to help restore or maintain a healthy moisture balance. Aloe is also know for its soothing properties and can help to relieve a dry and/or itchy scalp.

3. **Vitamin E** —Vitamin E oil is an all-natural, vegetable-derived preservative used in hair and body care products to prevent other oils from turning rancid. This lightweight ingredient is easily absorbed by the hair and is highly regarded for its moisturizing benefits.

4. **Jojoba Oil** — Jojoba oil is extracted from the seeds of the desert *shrub simondsia chinesis* and closely resembles the natural sebum produced by the scalp. This emollient helps to restore shine and manageability, without causing product build-up or leaving a sticky residue. Coconut, sunflower, and sweet almond oils are also great, all-natural moisturizing agents.

5. **Wheat Protein** — This highly refined, natural protein derived from whole wheat helps to improve body and impart shine to dry, distressed hair. This protein is often found in shampoos and conditioners formulated for damaged and/or color treated hair.

6. **Herbal Extracts** — Herbal extracts are frequently added to hair care products, albeit in small amounts, for their moisturizing or conditioning properties. Some common herbal extracts found in commercial shampoos are: rosemary, lavender, peppermint, calendula, and nettle.

7. **Glycerin** — Derived from palm oil, glycerin is a natural humectant and conditioning agent that helps your hair attract and retain moisture. This ingredient is easily absorbed by the hair shaft and frequently used in shampoos and conditioners to increase their moisturizing properties.

8. **Panthenol or Pro Vitamin B** — Panthenol is used in hair care

products to impart sheen, improve manageability, and replenish moisture. This Vitamin B complex has also been shown to increase the strength and thickness of hair, making it far more resistant to breakage, split ends, and damage caused by brushing, blow drying, chemical services, and other environmental factors.

9. **Cholesterol** — Cholesterol makes a wonderful addition to hair conditioners and helps to enhance luster, body, and softness to dry and brittle hair.

10. **Lecithin** — From the Greek word meaning "egg yolk"; this natural antioxidant, emollient, and emulsifier is used in a variety of cosmetic preparations. Note: egg yolk is 8 - 9% lecithin.

"Natural" *Beware*

Consumers eager to make healthy choices often err in thinking that shampoos which come in environmentally friendly packaging with the words "all-natural" or "organic" on the labels are safe for washing their *185* hair. In reality, many of these "natural" shampoos cost three times as much as everyday brands, yet contain the same harmful ingredients as most commercial shampoos. One only need read the labels carefully to find potentially harmful synthetic preservatives, cheap texture enhancing additives, chemically-derived sudsing agents, and artificial colorants and fragrances.[26] Because there is no official legal definition for the word "natural", we must start protecting ourselves and our pocketbooks from false claims and empty promises. Here are some common examples to be on the look out for:

- *Natural:* is a word that suggests a product's ingredients are derived from natural sources (i.e. plants or animals) as opposed to being manufactured synthetically. Unfortunately, the fine print sometimes reveals that this is not always the case.

- *Organic:* the use of this term implies that a product contains all-natural ingredients and no synthetic additives. But do a quick-check of the ingredient list and you may be surprised to discover artificial additives are still present.

- *Hypoallergenic:* sounds so scientific, doesn't it? All it means is that a product is less likely to cause an allergic reaction -- but there are no uniform standards for substantiating this claim. Similarly, the terms "dermatologist-tested", "sensitivity tested", "allergy tested", or "nonirritating" do not offer complete assurance that a product will not cause an allergic reaction.

- *Alcohol Free:* usually means the product doesn't contain ethyl alcohol (or grain alcohol). Still, many cosmetics are labeled "alcohol free" -- yet still contain fatty alcohols, such as cetyl, stearyl, cetearyl, or lanolin.

- *Fragrance Free:* suggests a product has no detectable odor. In reality, products advertised as such may contain fragrance additives to disguise the offensive odors of raw materials. They can still be labeled fragrance free, so long as the final product doesn't impart a discernible scent.

- *Cruelty Free:* implies that final product has not been tested on animals. However, this claim doesn't ensure that the raw materials used in the manufacturing process were not tested on our cute furry friends.

Many companies spend tons of money – hiring clever PR/ advertising execs to create slick campaigns and lots of spin so that the public assumes that the products they're buying are safe. While it's nice to imagine that these corporations wouldn't knowingly market products with questionable impact on the public's health, it would also be naïve to believe everything a company lists on its packaging is absolutely true and perfectly safe. (Remember the whole cigarette debacle and how long it took for the truth to come out.)

In the meantime, the best defense is a good offense; read the labels and be cautiously skeptical. Follow the advice, caveat emptor, or in English, *Let the Buyer Beware.* By being informed, you can increase your chances of using the best and safest products.

For More Information

In addition to the information provided here, you can learn more about the various ingredients in your cosmetics from the following reference publications, available at most public libraries:

- *International Cosmetic Ingredient Dictionary and Handbook*, published by the Cosmetic, Toiletry, and Fragrance Association

- Paula Begoun. *Don't Go Shopping for Hair-Care Products Without Me: Over 4,000 Products Reviewed, Plus the Latest Hair-Care Information*

- Kim Erickson. *Drop-Dead Gorgeous: Protecting Yourself from the Hidden Dangers of Cosmetics*

- Aubrey Hampton. *What's In Your Cosmetics: A Complete Consumer's Guide To Natural & Synthetic Ingredients*

- David Steinman and Samuel S. Epstein. *The Safe Shopper's Bible: A Consumer's Guide to Nontoxic Household Products*

- Judi Vance. *Beauty to Die for: The Cosmetic Consequence*

- Ruth Winter. *A Consumer's Dictionary of Cosmetic Ingredients: Complete Information About the Harmful and Desirable Ingredients in Cosmetics*

Key Points to Remember

- You can protect yourself from natural imposters by learning to read the labels and recognizing the ingredients found on cosmetic packaging.

- What we put on our bodies is just as important as what we put in our bodies.

- Look for products, where natural items are at or near the top of the list of ingredients.

Chapter 15
In the Kitchen
Making Products at Home

Since the beginning of time, black women all over the globe have been whipping up recipes using natural ingredients to promote healthy hair growth. Shea butter, which comes from Western Africa, has been used for centuries by African women to condition and protect their hair from the sun. In ancient Egypt, where women frequently wore wigs and hair extensions, citrus juice and sweet almond oil were commonly used to cleanse the scalp and give the hair a fresh scent. To our sub-Saharan ancestors, the avocado was not only a tasty delicacy, but also an ingredient rich in nutrients great for treating scalp ailments and used as a deep conditioner. Although African beauty secrets have been a wonderful source of inspiration for manufacturers of modern day cosmetics, very few commercial products capture the pure essence of these ancient health remedies.

While we have come a long way thanks to advancements in technology, there are still many benefits to making your own hair care products. Plus, it's much easier than you think. If you can boil water and read directions, you'll have no problem following the simple recipes in this chapter! Not only is it cheaper to make your own hair care treatments, "but many of these recipes work just as well as, if not better than, expensive store brought brands," says Alisha Davis (AKA Motown Girl), whose popular natural hair care website www.motowngirl.com features many homemade hair care recipes in addition to those found here. Most of these recipes cost less than $2 to make and you can find many of the ingredients in your kitchen or at your local grocers or health food store. You can also relax and take comfort in knowing the ingredients you are using on your hair and body are 100% natural.

The recipes in this chapter do not contain any artificial preservatives or synthetic ingredients, so preparations containing perishable items should be refrigerated immediately. For your own benefit, it is usually a good idea to keep track of which ingredients you have used -- either by writing them down in a journal or on a label affixed to the jar containing the mixture. Most of these products/recipes also have a limited shelf life, so you'll want to keep a record of the dates when you made any treatment. Preparation is key, so set aside your ingredients beforehand.

It's always important to sterilize all containers and equipment before use. The can be done by placing your bowls and jars in a dishwasher or in boiling water (metal only) for fifteen to twenty minutes. Alternatively, you can use a solution made for sterilizing babies' bottles to disinfect your plastic jars and utensils. If you have sensitive skin or allergies, be sure to apply a small amount of product to your hand first to see how your skin reacts. If you experience any redness, swelling, itching or irritation, refrain from using the product again.

WARNING: The results of any of the homemade hair recipes contained in this chapter are not guaranteed and are for your own personal experimentation purposes. Each individual may react differently to an ingredient or a specific treatment. Accordingly, it is highly recommended that before using any recipe, you read the list of ingredients closely to determine if you have any allergies or any medical restrictions that prevent you from ingesting certain substances. Should you have any health care-related questions or concerns, please contact your physician or other health care provider.

190

Shampoos

Here are some simple and easy shampoo recipes to try at home. These shampoos are made with all natural ingredients. They provide gentle yet effective cleansing and will not strip your hair of its natural oils or leave it feeling dry and brittle.

Natural Hair Shampoo

- ½ cup water
- ¼ cup castile soap
- ½ tsp jojoba oil (if you have oily hair, omit this ingredient entirely or try using sesame oil instead)

Mix all the ingredients together and pour into a clean, squeeze bottle. Allow the mixture to sit overnight and thicken. Shampoo as you would normally and follow with a thorough, cool water rinse.

Natural Herbal Shampoo

- ½ cup water
- ½ cup burdock, lavender or sandalwood
- ½ cup Natural Hair Shampoo (see above)
- 2 tbsp glycerin

Combine water and herbs together and heat on low to make a strong tea. Let the mixture stand for at least thirty minutes before adding the shampoo and glycerin to the herbal water mixture. Stir well. Pour the final mixture into a clean squeeze bottle. Allow it to sit overnight, in order to thicken. Shampoo as you would ordinarily and follow with a cool water rinse.

Egg Shampoo

Raw egg is great for the hair and will give your mane major shine and body.

- 1 raw egg
- 1 tbsp Basic Shampoo

191

Combine all the ingredients in a bowl and whisk together until smooth. Use shampoo immediately and follow up with a cool water rinse. Do not use hot water or you will end up with scrambled eggs in your hair! Discard any remaining shampoo (since it is perishable).

Olive Oil Shampoo

Olive oil is famous for being a great conditioner. It can also help to make your hair stronger. Of course, if your hair is already oily, you'll want to reduce the amount of olive oil called for in this recipe. To make your shampoo more personal, add your own natural fragrance while you mix it up.

- ¼ cup olive oil
- 1 cup castile soap

Blend together all ingredients until the mixture has a smooth consistency. Pour the shampoo into a clean squeeze bottle with an airtight lid.

Shampoo as you would ordinarily and follow with a cool water rinse.

Dry Shampoo Recipe

Cornstarch is great for absorbing the scalp's oils and comes in handy if you are in a pinch. If your hair is naturally dry, remember that a little goes a long way.

- ¼ cup cornstarch

Sprinkle the cornstarch in your hair, let it absorb for a few minutes. Use a brush to remove. Rinse your brush after use.

Hair Rinses

Our hair and scalp can really suffer the damaging effects of all kinds of things -- some of which we can control, like hair dye and overly strong shampoos, and other factors that are beyond our control. When this happens, a simple and easy solution can be the application of a good, natural rinse -- which can retsore you hair's strength and healthy glow. Here are a few recipes you can try to restore shine and body to your hair. Make sure that you apply these rinses *after* you are done shampooing and that you do not rinse them from your hair. While these are called *rinses,* the name is slightly misleading. You are meant to rinse the shampoo out – but not the formula (rinse) you put on after shampooing.

MotownGirl's Lemon/Honey Rinse

- 2 tsp honey
- ¼ cup lemon juice
- 4 cups warm water

Combine in a large bowl and warm for fifteen to twenty seconds in a microwave. After shampooing and conditioning hair, pour mixture through hair. Do not rinse out. Dry as usual.

Honey Hair Shine

Not only does honey taste delicious -- but it can also restore body and shine to your hair.

- 1 tsp honey
- 4 cups warm water

Pour the honey into warm water. If you warm the honey a little, it's easier to pour and mix. Remember, this treatment is for use *after* shampooing. Douse your hair with your Honey Hair Shine and don't rinse it out! Then just dry your hair however you normally would and go out with a new glow!

Herbal Hair Rinse

- 1 cup distilled or spring water
- 5 - 6 tbsp of dried herbs (choose one to three herbs from the list below)
- ceramic or glass bowl or small pot
- plastic squeeze bottle
- small piece of un-dyed cheese cloth (optional)

Bring water to a boil and pour over your herbs. Since you don't want actual bits of herbs in your hair, you can use a small piece of un-dyed cheesecloth to make a little tea bag. Place the herbs in the center of the cheese cloth, gather the edges together, and then tie the bag closed with a knot or a small piece of string). Pour your herbal mix into the container that is used for steeping and cover. Allow the mixture to steep for ten to thirty minutes. The longer you allow the herbs to sit, the stronger the rinse. It's just like making tea! When it cools, you can pour the solution into a squeeze bottle for easy application.

After shampooing pour the "tea" over your hair and massage gently into your scalp. *Note:* This product doesn't have a long shelf life. In fact, this recipe only yields enough for one treatment.

Select two or three herbs from the list. Make sure you pick herbs that will help your own hair's specific condition and texture.

HERBS FOR DRY HAIR: Elderflower, clover, comfrey leaf, burdock, chamomile, lavender, rose, and sandalwood. These herbs not only encourage healthy hair, but they also smell great.

HERBS FOR OILY HAIR: Lemongrass, peppermint, quassia chips, rosemary, white willow bark, cedar wood, cypress, sage, and patchouli are great for oily hair and discourage the scalp from producing excess oil.

HERBS FOR DANDRUFF: Birch bark, nettle, peppermint, and white willow bark.

Conditioners

Here are some conditioners you can try for added shine and body. These natural conditioners not only smooth and detangle, but they also help to maintain your hair's natural moisture balance while minimizing breakage and split ends.

Natural Hair Conditioner

This recipe is great for those who live in cooler and dryer climates, where weather conditions can sometimes be rough on the hair and skin. Use this conditioner once a week to keep your hair soft, radiant, and the envy of all of your friends.

- 1 tsp almond oil
- 1 tsp avocado oil
- 1 tsp olive oil
- 1 egg yolk
- 1 tbsp honey
- 1 tbsp fresh lemon juice

Mix all the ingredients together in a bowl and stir thoroughly. You can use a fork, a whisk, or even a mixer to achieve a smooth consistency. This is a conditioner that is used before you shampoo. Massage the mixture into your mane and scalp then cover your hair with a plastic shower cap or plastic wrap for fifteen minutes. At the end of fifteen minutes, hop into the shower and shampoo. Rinse well. If you have any conditioner left over and no one to share it with, throw it away. This recipe doesn't keep long.

Rosemary Honey Hair Conditioner

Rosemary (Rosmarinus officinalis) is thought to stimulate hair growth and to be a great remedy for dandruff and itchy scalps. This easy recipe will leave your hair feeling softer, more manageable, and smelling wonderful. Warning: Avoid this recipe if you are pregnant, have high blood pressure, or are epileptic
.

- ½ cup honey
- ¼ cup warmed olive oil (2 tbsp for normal to oily hair)
- 4 drops essential oil of rosemary
- 1 tsp xanthum gum (available in health food stores)

195

Place all the ingredients into a small bowl and mix thoroughly. Pour into a clean, plastic bottle with a tight-fitting lid. Apply a small amount at a time to slightly dampened hair. Massage scalp and work mixture through hair until completely coated. Cover hair with a warm towel (towel can be heated in a microwave or dryer) or shower cap for thirty minutes. Remove towel or shower cap; shampoo lightly and rinse with cool water. Dry as normal and enjoy softer, shinier hair the natural way.

Herbal Egg Conditioner

- 2 tsps lemon juice
- 1 tsp honey
- 1 egg
- 3 drops rosemary oil
- 1/4 cup almond or coconut oil

Beat lemon juice, honey, and egg together. Pour mixture into a double boiler and heat. Stir until warm and creamy. Let cool. Combine rosemary oil and vegetable oil and add slowly to egg mixture. Mix well. Massage into clean, damp hair. Cover hair with a warm towel or shower cap for thirty minutes. Remove towel or shower cap and rinse with cool water.

Honey/Olive Oil Conditioner

The extreme cold (outside) and heat (artificial/inside) we endure throughout winter can make even the greatest hair look (and feel) like straw. This nourishing conditioner blends honey for shine and olive oil for moisture to make your hair softer and shinier. This treatment is a little sticky, but well worth it. Don't worry – it rinses out easily.

- ½ cup honey
- ¼ cup olive oil (2 tbsp for normal hair)

Mix the honey and olive oil together. Work a small amount at a time through hair until coated. Cover hair with shower cap. Leave on for thirty minutes. Remove shower cap. Shampoo well and rinse. Dry as normal.

Protein-Rich, Nourishing Conditioner

This recipe strengthens the hair and restores softness, shine, and manageability to damaged hair.

- 1 egg white
- 5 tbsp plain yogurt

Beat egg white until foamy. Gently add in the plain yogurt. Apply to your hair in small sections and leave on for ten to fifteen minutes. Rinse and follow up with a moisturizing, deep conditioner for wonderful results! Style as usual.

MotownGirl's Caribbean Queen Conditioner

This recipe was given to MotownGirl by a close friend whose family has used this treatment for generations to protect their hair from the warm climate and bright sun of the West Indies.

- 2 eggs
- 1 tbsp olive oil

- 1 tbsp vegetable glycerin
- ½ cup purified water
- 1 tsp apple cider vinegar

Combine all ingredients and whisk thoroughly. After shampooing, massage conditioner through your hair and cover with a plastic shower cap. Leave on for at least fifteen to twenty minutes. Rinse thoroughly.

MotownGirl's Leave-In Conditioner

This treatment will give your hair a nice sheen and help enhance curl definition. It also has a pleasant smell -- depending on which oils you use for fragrance.

- 8 oz. pump bottle
- 1 cup conditioner
- 1/8 cup oil (avocado, coconut or olive oil)
- 1 tbs vegetable glycerin
- 1 tbs silk amino acid
- fragrance oil for scent (optional). Here are some examples you could use: apple, vanilla, pina colada, strawberry, or even mango! You can purchase these online at www.fromnaturewithlove.com or at your local Whole Foods Supermarket.

197

Combine ingredients together and pour into pump bottle. Shake well. The consistency should be somewhat thick. For best results, apply to damp hair. You don't need to use much! A little goes a long way.

This recipe works best with thick, heavy conditioners like Suave Humectant, Eluence, or Pantene Hydrating Curls. Double up the recipe as needed and substitute ingredients (such as different oils or fragrances) to suit your own, personal taste.

Tropical Conditioner

Avocado is recommended for its hydrating benefits and proteins. Of course there are other fruits (e.g. banana, papaya, or mango) that you can use for your natural hair treatment, using the same instructions as above.

- 1 avocado (peeled and mashed)
- 1 cup coconut milk

Combine mashed avocado with coconut milk. Mash together until mixture is smooth and has the consistency of conditioner. Comb through the hair and let sit for – ten to fifteen minutes. Wash out. If your hair is long, divide into several sections and apply the mixture near your roots first and then proceed to massage the paste down towards your ends. For deeper conditioning, place a hot, damp towel around your head or cover your head with a shower cap. *Warning:* Avoid this recipe if you are pregnant, have high blood pressure, or are epileptic.

Mayonnaise Hair Pack

This recipe is great for dry hair and will leave your tresses feeling soft and looking beautiful. Note, you can also make your own mayonnaise by mixing one egg with one cup of virgin olive oil.

- ½ cup mayonnaise

Apply mayonnaise to dry hair. Work into hair really well and then cover with a plastic bag. Allow to set for fifteen minutes. Rinse thoroughly and then shampoo as usual. *Special Note:* Make sure to use mayonnaise and NOT salad dressing, which will dry your hair out.

Clarifying Treatments

Unlike commercial clarifying shampoos, which use strong detergents, these all-natural treatments will remove buildup left on your scalp without stripping your hair of its natural oils.

Basic Clarifying Treatment

- 2 cups warm water
- ½ cup lemon juice

Mix ingredients together and massage through damp hair. Let treatment sit for ten minutes. Rinse, condition, and style as usual. This recipe will leave the hair clean and smelling great! *Note:* This treatment doesn't produce great results if you frequently use heavy oils and petroleum based styling products.

Baking Soda Clarifying Treatment

Use this mixture if your hair is starting to feel yucky; it will help get rid of extra build-up. This treatment will give your hair that clean feeling without stripping it of its natural oils. If your hair is long or thick, you can double or even triple the ingredients. One tablespoon of baking soda may not seem like a lot -- but DO NOT add more unless you add more water. Your hair WILL become hard and brittle...trust me!

- 1 tbsp baking soda
- 1 ½ cup warm water

Combine ingredients in a cup or spray bottle. The mixture should be liquidy...NOT gritty. Spray the solution onto your hair and work *199* through your mane. Leave on for two to three minutes, then rinse.

Apple Cider Vinegar Rinse

Vinegar rinses can do wonders for the hair! They are great at removing the residue and build-up left on the hair that come with regular use of styling products, which cause the hair to look and feel dull and lifeless. Vinegar also cuts through excess oils, which sometimes give the hair a waxy feeling. The result is soft and shiny hair that is manageable and has tons of body.

- cup apple cider vinegar
- 1 cup water

Mix ingredients together and use as a final rinse after shampooing. Be sure to distribute this mixture throughout your hair evenly for complete coverage. Leave on for two to three minutes and then rinse with cold water. What a cinch! Use bi-weekly as a hair clarifying treatment. Take care to avoid getting this treatment in your eyes. It does sting.

Miscellaneous

Here are some additional beauty recipes made from natural ingredients that you can try at home for gorgeous, lustrous hair:

Whipped Shea Butter Pomade

- 4 oz. of unrefined shea butter
- ¼ cup of sweet almond oil
- ⅛ cup of castor oil
- 1 Vitamin E capsule
- 5 drops of ylang ylang
- 3 drops of vanilla

Melt shea butter over low heat using the double-boiler method. When the shea butter melts completely, stir in the sweet almond oil and castor oil and allow to cool. Once the mixture has a soft butter consistency, break open a Vitamin E capsule and squeeze its contents into the mixture. Beat on low with an electric mixer that is outfitted with whisks until the mix becomes fluffy and has the appearance of egg whites. Add in ylang-ylang and vanilla for fragrance. Pour into plastic container and let cool. This treatment has a nice thick and creamy consistency and smells good enough to eat.

Note, improper heating of shea butter can cause the butter to crystallize as it cools. To avoid this, shea butter should be heated to about 175 degrees and kept at that temperature for at least twenty minutes. This will allow the butter to melt completely and will prevent crystals from forming after the butter has cooled.

Rosemary Hair Oil

- 2 tbsp dried rosemary
- ½ cup olive oil

Combine rosemary and olive oil in a bowl. Heat in the microwave on high for two minutes or on the stovetop on low. Do not allow to boil. Once the mixture has cooled completely, let stand for two to three days in order to give the oil the chance to absorb the essential ingredients from the rosemary. Pour the solution through a funnel lined with a coffee filter to remove any solids. Transfer the remains into a clean bottle. Use by massaging a small amount in your scalp after shampooing or before going to bed at night. *Special Note:* For dry and damaged hair, substitute jojoba oil for the olive oil. For oilier hair, replace olive oil with sesame oil.

Brown Sugar Scalp Scrub

- 1 tbs brown sugar
- 3 tbs Natural Hair Conditioner

Mix ingredients together. Apply to damp scalp and gently massage in a circular motion. Rinse well, then shampoo.

MotownGirl's Homemade Spritz

If you find that your hair doesn't respond well to oils or hair butters, try this mixture for softness and mucho moisture! This recipe is also great for touching up puffs, twists, and braids.

201

- 3 oz. distilled water
- 1 oz. of a light conditioner (Suave, White Rain etc.)
- ½ oz. oil (olive oil, avocado, grape seed, or sweet almond oil)

Pour ingredients into spray bottle and shake well. Spritz hair lightly. Do not rinse out.

MotownGirl's Hair Growth Mixture

- ¼ cup pure Vitamin E oil
- ¼ cup castor or jojoba oil
- 15 drops rosemary oil
- 15 drops peppermint oil

Place ingredients in container and stir well. Pour a quarter-size amount into your palm and apply to your scalp and the area around your temples. Massage gently. Using this treatment several times a week is acceptable as long as you wash your hair frequently (e.g. every seven to ten days).

MotownGirl's Egg & Honey Treatment

In this recipe, the honey smoothes and softens the hair while the egg and almond oil penetrate and moisturize the hair shaft.

- 1 tbsp honey
- 1 egg yolk
- ½ tsp almond oil
- 1 tbsp yogurt

Mix ingredients together. Apply to hair and let sit for thirty minutes. Rinse well, then style as usual.

Hot Oil Treatment for Dry Hair

Olive oil is one of those all-purpose remedies that is great for almost anything – your hair, your scalp, your nails, and your skin. This natural moisturizer will also repair split ends, heal dandruff, and give your hair a silky and shiny appearance.

212

- ¼ to ½ cup olive oil

Heat oil in the microwave on medium for approximately one to two minutes. For easy application, carefully pour the olive oil into a spray bottle and apply to the ends and dry parts of your hair. Avoid getting oil onto your scalp. Cover your head with a shower cap or a warm towel for at least thirty minutes. Rinse and then shampoo and condition as usual. For extra conditioning, some naturals advise sleeping with olive oil on your hair and washing it out the next morning.

MotownGirl's Egg & Olive Oil Hair Treatment

Although easy to prepare, this treatment can be somewhat messy. But the results do make the effort worthwhile.

- 2 eggs
- 4 tbsp of olive oil

Mix well and smooth through your hair. Cover head with shower cap.

Let treatment sit on hair for ten minutes. Rinse well, then shampoo. Dry hair and style as usual.

MotownGirl's Scalp Energizer

Give yourself a real scalp refresher with this energizing treatment.

- 2 drops pure peppermint oil
- 4 oz water

Place ingredients in spray bottle and apply directly to scalp. Shake well before use. This mixture will leave your scalp feeling fresh and smelling great!

Homemade Hair Gel

- 1 cup water
- 2 tbs. flax seed
- 2 drops scented essential oil of your choice

213

Combine water and seeds in a small saucepan. Bring to a boil and remove from heat. Allow mixture to sit for thirty minutes. Strain through a fine colander or coffee filter. When completely cooled, add the scented oil of your choice. Transfer to a wide-mouthed jar with lid. Use as you would any hair gel product.

Dandruff Treatments

Dandruff is a fairly common scalp condition, characterized by excessive shedding of dry flaky skin. Improper hair care, poor diet, stress, fatigue and genetics, among other factors, are all causes of this condition. For serious cases of dandruff -- or if your condition doesn't improve-- consult your physician or dermatologist.

For Oily, Flaky Scalp

- 2 tbsp apple cider vinegar of fresh lemon juice
- 2 tbsp distilled water
- 2 tbsp olive oil

Mix all ingredients together and massage into your scalp. Leave on for twenty minutes before shampooing.

For Dry, Flaky Scalp

- 2 tbsp jojoba oil
- ¼ tbsp tea tree oil

Blend the two oils together and massage into wet hair. Leave on for ten minutes, then shampoo out.

214

Key Points to Remember

- Many homemade recipes work just as well, if not better than, expensive store-bought brands.

- Preparation is key.

- Keep records of when you make treatment(s) to prevent spoilage.

- Always do a skin test before using any product.

215

The sky is the limit when it comes to trying different homemade recipes. The mixtures listed here are just a starting point. You should feel free to experiment with different ingredients until you discover what your hair likes and responds to best. Sometimes, you'll stumble upon the ideal treatments when you are creative and willing to try new things. If you are the adventurous type, try substituting juices, teas, or milks when a recipe calls for water -- or add a few drops of honey or olive oil when the recipe doesn't require it. The added nutritional benefits are a huge bonus and your hair and body will thank you for it.

Additional Resources

The following books and websites offer more information on making your own skin and hair care preparations using all natural ingredients.

Books

Earthly Bodies & Heavenly Hair: Natural and Healthy Personal Care for Every Body. Dina Falconi. Ceres Press 1997.

Making Natural Liquid Soaps: Herbal Shower Gels/Conditioning Shampoos/ Moisturizing Hand Soaps. Catherine Failor. Storey Publishing, LLC 2000.

Natural Beauty at Home. More than 200 Easy - To- Use Recipes for Body, Bath and Hair. Janice Cox. Henry Holt 1994.

Natural Beauty for All Seasons. 250 Simple Recipes and Gift-Giving Ideas for Year-Round Beauty. Janice Cox. Henry Holt 1996.

Natural Beauty from the Garden. More than 200 Do-It-Yourself Beauty Recipes and Garden Idea. Janice Cox. Henry Holt 1999.

Natural Body Basics: Making Your Own Cosmetics. Dorie Byers. Gooseberry Hill 1996.

Websites

http://www.fromnaturewithlove.com

http://www.motowngirl.com

http://www.nappturality.com

http://www.pioneerthinking.com

http://www.thesage.com

Ready-Made Products

If you're short on time, but still want the benefits of using hair care preparations made with natural ingredients, the following companies manufacture products that are either 100% natural or contain a limited amount of synthetic additives:

Aubrey Organics
http://www.aubrey-organics.com/index.cfm

217

Aveda
http://www.aveda.com

Black Earth Products
http://www.naturalhair.org
http://www.blackearthproducts.com

Jane's Carter Solution
http://www.janecartersolution.com

Nature's Gate
http://www.natures-gate.com

New Bein'
http://www.newbein.com

Oyin Homemade
http://oyinhomemade.com

Chapter 16

Hair Loss

Getting to the Root of the Problem

I have a confession to make. Once upon a time, I curled my hair too often, wore my braids too tight, and put a weave in when I knew my strands needed a break. After coming to the realization that my hairline might never grow back, I put an end to the vicious cycle of abusing my edges, then begging for their forgiveness. As black women, we take great pride in styling our hair -- but we're all guilty of hair abuse. Unfortunately, harsh styling practices have left many of us with severe breakage, receding hairlines, and permanent hair loss. Sometimes, the problem can be fixed with a simple change in hairstyle or styling technique. Yet, at other times the issue reflects a more serious, underlying condition that requires medical attention.

Al· o· pe· cia

Alopecia, the medical term for hair loss, has become a serious issue for black women. "I see at least five patients a day with this concern -- and that number is growing," says Dr. Susan Taylor of Dermatology Hill in Philadelphia, PA. Although this condition takes many forms, black women are prone to breakage, thinning hair (*traction alopecia*), and complete hair loss due to unhealthy styling practices (*follicular degeneration syndrome*).

In most cases, chemical relaxers are the primary culprit. Years of chemical relaxing can cause irreversible damage to the scalp and hair follicles, resulting in permanent hair loss. "Tight braids, ponytails, and bonding glue are also to blame," says Gerry Mayo, hair restoration expert and owner of Endless Creations of You Hair Salon in Upper Darby, PA. Many of Mayo's clients fall victim to what she calls the "*double whammy*." "Black women are destroying their hair when they put the weaves and braids in -- and pulling their hair out when they take the extensions down." To eliminate this problem, Mayo recommends seeking out a skilled professional, who is knowledgeable about hair extensions and understands the proper technique for their removal.

For many women, the day-to-day stress caused by balancing the responsibilities of work and family is a major cause of hair loss. Genetics may also be a factor. Still, Dr. Taylor is quick to point out that "inherited genes play a small part in very few cases." In most instances, hair loss can be traced back to unhealthy styling practices and/or changes in hormone levels. Excessive heat from blow-drying, curling, or pressing the hair can take a toll on healthy tresses too. Fluctuations in your hormones -- caused by pregnancy, menopause, poor nutrition, surgery, illness, or certain medications -- can also trigger hair loss.

Alopecia areata is another form of hair loss, which causes the hair follicles on the scalp and other parts of the body to stop producing hair. People who have this type of alopecia develop small dime or quarter-sized round bald spots on the scalp or other hair-bearing parts of the body. Although the exact cause of alopecia areata remains unknown, many individuals who suffer from this condition, including Milwaukee Bucks forward Charlie Villanueva, are in perfect health and still lead normal, active lives.

When to See a Doctor

Valerie Winston's story begins like so many hair loss patients who notice their hair thinning near the front of the scalp and in the crown area. Her stylist initially attributed the loss to stress and tried adding a few pieces to give her style more fullness -- but this proved to be a temporary solution. "I even tried Rogaine," says the 41-year-old banker, "but nothing seemed to help." After months passed -- and her condition got progressively worse -- Winston sought medical treatment. Her doctor diagnosed her with *hyperthyroidism* and attributed the hair loss to this condition. Thanks to early treatment and detection, she says, "I was able to save both my hair and my life."

It's definitely normal to shed between 100-125 hairs per day. If, however, you start to notice excessive amounts of hair in your brush, on your clothing, or in the shower, there may be cause for concern. Don't bother wasting your time on the SuperGro hair care products found at your local beauty supply store. "Most of these products are ineffective and contain petroleum and mineral oil, which clog your pores and slow hair growth," says Dr. Taylor. Your best bet is to make an appointment to see a dermatologist, who can help you to identify the cause of your hair loss and determine the most effective course of treatment. Hair loss due to use of chemical relaxers, bonding glue, or tight braids is frequently misdiagnosed by individuals who are unfamiliar with the styling practices of African-American women. So if possible, seek the opinion of a professional who is familiar with black hair.

Many black women make the mistake of ignoring their symptoms until their hair loss is in the advanced or final stages -- often blaming stress, the brand of relaxer, or other factors for their condition. Waiting too long to seek treatment makes stimulating new hair growth and preventing further hair loss extremely difficult -- and may even jeopardize your overall health if this condition is an early sign of a serious medical illness. For this reason, it is always best to seek professional, medical attention sooner rather than later.

Root Causes of Hair Loss

Alopecia may be triggered by several different factors, including:

- Misuse of chemical relaxers, permanent hair dyes, or other chemical processes, which may include not following directions and using products in dangerous combinations *211*

- Excessive pulling from various hairstyle including, braids, rollers, weaves, and ponytails, and long heavy locks

- Excessive heat from blow dryers, hot combs, curling irons, and electric rollers

- Hormonal fluctuations due to normal life processes (e.g. menstrual cycles, stress, responses to birth controls pills or hormone therapy)

- Hypothyroidism or hyperthyroidism

- Chronic illness like HIV/AIDS, lupus, mono, or auto-immune deficiency

- Anemia caused by very severe iron-deficiency

- Fungal infection/ringworm

- Bacterial infection of the hair follicles -- known as folliculitis

- Severe fever or prolonged infection

- Surgery

- Low-protein diet

- Sudden, dramatic weight change

- Medication interaction or response

- Chemotherapy

- Extreme Stress

Treating Hair Loss

Understanding the nature of your condition is the first step towards remedying the problem. In some instances, hair loss is temporary and treatment may not be required. In other cases, medication, hair replacement surgery, hairpieces, or change in diet may offer effective treatment. Each has its advantages and disadvantages, which are more fully described below.

Rogaine

Women who experience thinning throughout the top of the head or the crown may benefit from the use of either a prescription or an over-the counter version of Rogaine. At this time, Rogaine is the only hair loss medication approved by the FDA for use by women. It can take three to four months to see results and up to six months to determine whether Rogaine will have any significant impact. Hair loss, however, will recur unless the product is used consistently. Rogaine is expensive, but Headwway, the generic version, makes this topical treatment more affordable.

Hair Transplants

Due to major breakthroughs and advancements in technology, hair transplants now produce natural looking results, which even the most seasoned hair stylist can't detect. This minor outpatient surgery involves a simple procedure, which relocates bald resistant follicles to areas of the scalp where your hair is thinning. Hair-transplants can be expensive and may require multiple surgeries. This procedure may also result in minor scarring and carries a slight risk of infection. Despite the potential drawbacks, this procedure has an extremely high success rate and yields excellent results, which can last a lifetime. For more information about hair transplants or to locate a doctor in your area who specializes in this procedure, visit the www.hairtransplantnetwork.com.

Hair Pieces

Hair weaves and wigs can also help to camaflouge hair loss and improve the overall appearance of thinning hair. Hair pieces are a safe and affordable option. However, they're no substitute for seeing your doctor. If you're considering this option, be sure to check with your physician first in order to rule out a medical condition.

Scalp Pencils

You can purchase a scalp pencil form your local beauty supply store to fill in bald spots or disguise a receding hairline. Fill in sparse areas with a freshly-sharpened scalp pencil by drawing light, short strokes in the direction of hair growth.

Natural Alternatives

Diet and nutrition can also be an effective remedy for treating alopecia. Some studies have shown that vitamins may help to prevent and/or reduce hair loss. Many nutritionists and health experts actually believe that Americans have the greatest incidence of baldness due to our unhealthy eating habits. If you prefer a more holistic approach, the following natural remedies may prove effective in minimizing hair loss:

- *Get adequate protein.* Hair is composed mostly of protein, so you'll want to eat a well-balanced diet rich in this ingredient to help reduce and/or prevent further hair loss. Chicken and fish are excellent sources of protein and other essential nutrients. Other good sources of protein include eggs, beans, and yogurt.

- *Increase your iron in-take.* Due to a decrease in iron levels, anemia is also a common cause of hair loss in women. If you are anemic, be sure to eat plenty of iron-rich foods – such as lean red meat, whole grain cereals, dark green leafy vegetables, eggs, dates, and raisins to promote hair growth and reduce shedding.

- *Stock up on Vitamin A.* If hair loss is due to a thyroid condition, make sure you eat more foods rich in vitamin A and iodine. Carrots, spinach, walnuts, pumpkin seeds, and sea salt are rich sources of Vitamin A. If your iodine levels are low, turnips, cabbage, mustard, soybeans, peanuts, and pine nuts can also serve as supplements for this natural ingredient. But be careful. If your thyroid activity is normal, supplements high in vitamin A can actually accelerate hair loss.

- *Take Vitamin B6.* Vitamin B may also help to reduce hair shedding. For best results, eat foods rich in B vitamins -- such as beans, peas, carrots, cauliflower, soybeans, bran, nuts, and eggs.

- *Increase your estrogen levels.* Black cohosh is a medicinal herb used by women as a natural alternative to estrogen replacement. Some women have found that this supplement reduces hot flashes and minimizes hair loss due to fluctuations in their hormones caused by the onset of menopause.

Before treating hair loss with natural remedies, always be sure to consult with your physician to make sure that it doesn't interfere with your general health or any pre-existing medical condition.

Tips for Avoiding Hair Loss

If you have never experienced hair loss, then consider yourself lucky. An estimated two-thirds of women suffer from some form of hair loss during the course of their lives. If you have survived this ordeal or suffer from thinning strands, here are a few tips to help you prevent hair loss and maintain healthy tresses:

- If your hair loss is due to small braids, long weaves, or tight ponytails, you may need to change your hairstyle. If the hair loss is minimal, you may consider wearing larger braids, shorter weaves, and/or looser styles. Giving your hair and scalp a break from harsh styling practices can also help to relieve inflammation and will allow your scalp and hair time to heal.

- Black women often pull their hair too tightly to make their edges appear smoother or straighter in a ponytail or bun. Instead, try using hair gel or curl wax and tying a scarf around your head. This technique will give you the same results and help cut down on the stress and tension on your hairline.

- Eliminate or cut back on smoking, caffeine, and alcohol – all of which may rob the body of important nutrients and stunt your maximum hair-growing potential.

- Exercise caution when using heated styling appliances and pomades together to prevent melted pomade from coming in contact with the scalp. This practice can cause severe damage to the hair follicles and may lead to scarring and/or permanent hair loss.

- Limit your exposure to high heat or harsh chemical styling practices, such as coloring, straightening, perming, highlighting, or blow-drying the hair excessively -- which will only aggravate your condition further.

- Finally, give yourself a weekly scalp massage or get someone wonderful to do it for you. Therapeutic massages can increase circulation, reduce stress, and aid in promoting hair growth. Plus, it just feels sooo good!

Hair loss can be an emotionally traumatic experience. While you may feel embarrassed and alone, please rest assured that millions of women deal with this issue, even though it's not a topic of frequent discussion. The good news is that with early detection, most cases can be effectively treated. Before seeking a remedy or solution, consult with your doctor to determine the cause of your condition. In the meantime, keep your spirits up and try to maintain a positive attitude. Taking one day at a time and having an optimistic outlook can make a huge difference in your condition and greatly increase your chances for hair re-growth. For more information about treating or preventing hair loss, visit www.drsusantaylor.net and www.societyhilldermatology.com

Key Points to Remember

- Alopecia has become a serious problem among black women due to unhealthy styling practices.

- Avoid chemical services, excessive heat styling, and pulling your hair too tightly.

- With early detection, hair loss can often be effectively treated.

217

Epilouge

Naturally Ever After

This book is the culmination of many years of exhaustive but exhilarating research – and has proved to be quite a rewarding experience for me on many levels: personal, professional, and spiritual. I sincerely hope that you not only find yourself able to laugh, cry, and triumph with me through this work of self-discovery, but it is my wish that through my experiences, you are also able to identify with and ultimately understand that self-acceptance truly is the first step towards happiness.

At the beginning of this journey, I felt that the process of going natural was purely an aesthetic one. How it would look, how it would impact my style, how those around me would react…these seemed to be the questions that were of primary concern. As I look back, I realize that the importance of this decision had so little to do with my physical appearance and much more to do with accepting who I was, and not being ashamed by my defining characteristics as a black woman.

For too long, I bought into the myth that straight hair was somehow superior to my own – and spent hours and hours trying (without much success) to somehow obtain this artificial standard of beauty. I can't begin *229* to tell you how many years I spent crimping, ironing, gelling and perming my naps into submission. If only I had known then what I know now – that being natural is liberating and attractive in a whole different way!

I know what you're thinking – going natural is too drastic a step. Or, maybe one has to be a gorgeous supermodel to turn away from relaxers and accept the natural lifestyle. However, I am living proof that this is not the case! Sure, people often tell me how wonderful my hair looks, now that I've gone natural. But trust me, my kinks are far from perfect – and I wouldn't have it any other way. This process has not only helped me to come to grips with the insecurities that I have with my hair (and other parts of my body), but to realize that I don't need to keep buying into the damaging and consuming expectation of appearance. I only wish that I had learned earlier that I was focused on the superficial concept of beauty for too long – and that I was getting in the way of my own achievements and sense of personal happiness.

While compiling all the resources, data, and testimonials, I have met and spoken with thousands of women, who have shared their own, similar personal experiences and obstacles with me. And while this is heartwarming on one level – that we all share this bond– it's also frustrating to realize that so many of us are still struggling with these issues to this day.

It's been nearly three hundred years since we were brought over from Africa and we've lost a lot of our own heritage since then. But it's time for black women to reclaim our culture – and start taking pride in our amazing innate qualities and attributes. Moreover, given what we know about the risks and dangers of chemicals and other toxic substances, it's time to let go of the relaxers! They are probably causing all sorts of serious health issues -- and killing our spirits in the long run.

I'll admit, the journey can seem quite daunting at first, but I promise you that this important and essential decision will be on that you'll never regret. As you embark down the path to becoming a more complete, happier woman, you'll soon discover what it means to be the real you. Trust me --- this bold and rewarding lifestyle choice will translate and effect every aspect of your life and your hair will thank you for it! So set your curls free, enjoy one of your greatest beauty asset, and shout with me: THANK GOD I'M NATURAL!

221

Natural Hair
FAQs

General

I am graduating from college this spring and have decided to go natural. I'm thinking about wearing a TWA, but wanted to know if you think I'll have a hard time finding a job in corporate America.

Well, let me tell you, after wearing a wig for two years to keep my supervisors and colleagues happy, I realized that my hair didn't make much of a difference. At the end of the day, my wig didn't get me promoted or land me juicy assignments. So, my best advice would be to *be yourself.* Your future employer shouldn't have a problem with your hair, so long as it is neat and well groomed. This may sound cliché, but if you do good work, people will focus on your performance and not your hairstyle. If you ever get the vibe that a prospective employer is not feeling your style, trust your gut and keep your job search moving.

I'm thinking about going natural, but I don't want to be labeled as the "black panther" type. Any advice?

During the Civil Rights Era, being natural or wearing an Afro was seen as a political symbol. Today, wearing a natural is more of a fashion statement than a political one. Turn on the TV or flip through the pages of Essence and Vogue and you'll find neo-soul types like Jill Scott and Erykah Badu, cover models like Chrystelle Saint-Louis Augustin, and "conscious" role models such as Maya Angelou and Alice Walker, all sporting naturals. Despite their different styles, the one thing they all have in common is confidence. Truth be told, you can't be natural without it.

OK, I've been wearing a weave for six years. I see a lot of beautiful women with natural hair, but I'm scared that if I go natural I will have a hard time getting a date.

Trust me, you'll have no problem getting a date. As a matter of fact, some naturals find that they get more attention when they are natural than when they were relaxed. In my own experience, I can't tell you how many guys come up to me and want to touch my Afro puff or love the way my frizzy curls blow in the wind. For most guys, it's a breath of fresh hair to see a woman proudly rocking the hair she was born with!

Where can I find a natural salon in my area?

A list of salons catering to women with natural hair living in the U.S. and abroad can be found on my website www.thankgodimnatural.com or in the Salon Directory at the end of the book. You can also do a search on the Internet or ask friends and family members for a referral.

Relaxers

Why do relaxers cause my hair to break off?

Chemical relaxers change the pH of your hair, which can make it dry and brittle. This chemical service also causes the hair to lose it's elasticity -- thereby making it susceptible to breakage and damage. This is one of the primary reasons why you see so few black women with long relaxed hair.

If I get a kiddie perm or a texturizer am I still natural?

No! Kiddie perms and texturizers still contain chemicals that alter the pH and molecular structure of your hair. Although the concentration of chemicals in these products is sometimes lower than normal relaxers, they can still leave your hair weak and damaged.

Is it true that vinegar can take out your relaxer?

No. Once you use a relaxer, there is nothing you can do to reverse the process. The only way to go natural is to cut your relaxed hair off.

Are relaxers dangerous to my health?

Unfortunately, many of us have learned first-hand that relaxers can cause hair loss, hair breakage, hair-thinning, and scalp damage. In addition, these chemicals can be absorbed by the skin and transported through the bloodstream, where they may have an effect on the body's internal systems and organs. The FDA currently ranks chemical relaxers and hair dyes among its top consumer complaint areas. Despite these obvious dangers, relaxers are still sold to consumers and are considered "safe" by manufacturers for use at home.

Transitioning

I've been transitioning for six months wearing a bun and now my hair is starting to break. What should I do?

At this point, you basically have two options. You can continue to transition wearing protective styles like braids and cornrows -- or you can do *The Big Chop*. In your case, the Big Chop may be the best option. You should have at least 2-3" of new growth at this point, so there are plenty of hairstyles to choose from. Plus, your hair will thank you for letting go of those straggly, relaxed ends. Just remember, you can't serve two masters. Let go of the past and focus on your natural future.

I'm tired of wearing my hair pulled back into a bun. What other styles can I wear while I transition that won't damage my natural hair?

When transitioning, you'll want to look for a protective style that doesn't require a lot of manipulation. Try going for a twist out, a straw set, braids, cornrows, or maybe a weave. These styles don't require you to comb and brush your hair on a daily basis and will give your natural hair the chance to rest and grow into its own. For more information about protective styles, check out Chapter 7 – In The Pursuit of Nappiness.

Caring for Your Natural Hair

How often should I wash my hair?

Washing your hair at least once a week is highly recommended and also helps to keep your mane soft and moisturized.

I see lanolin and petroleum listed as ingredients on a lot of products. Are these good for my hair?

If you're looking for moisture, then you'll want to avoid products containing lanolin and petroleum. They both coat your strands and make it difficult for the hair to absorb water. Instead, go for products containing natural oils, like sweet almond, jojoba, and sunflower oil. Remember to scan the ingredient list carefully. Natural oils should be listed among the first few ingredients on the label. If the natural oils are listed at the very end, the product only contains trace amounts of these ingredients and won't have much of an effect.

What kind of hairbrush works best on natural hair?

Hands down, the Denman brush is by far the best styling tool for detangling wet hair. If you're looking to wear your hair pulled back into a bun with smooth edges, then a brush with soft boar's bristles will get the job done.

How often should I deep condition my hair?

You should deep condition your hair at least once a week. A good deep conditioner is usually thick and creamy. My personal favorite is Aveda Damage Remedy Intensive Restructuring Treatment. For best results, cover your head with a shower cap and sit under the dryer for fifteen to twenty minutes.

A lot of manufacturers like Pantene and Suave are making shampoos for women with natural hair. Can I trust these products?

In recent years, there has been a surge in products designed for women with natural hair. However, don't be fooled into thinking that just because a product comes in a brown bottle or has a red, black and green label that it's good for your hair. Everyone's hair type and texture is different. Experimenting with different brands is the only way to determine which products work best for you. There are also a number of homemade recipes that you can whip up for your hair. You can find many of them in Chapter 15 – Making Products at Home. So, experiment and have fun!

I just cut my hair, why is it so dry and hard?

Years of relaxing can damage your hair follicles. Remember, these little guys produce the natural oils that keep your hair soft and moisturized. As your hair follicles heal, they'll start to produce more of the natural oil that keeps your strands feeling soft and supple. Many naturals refer to the dry and brittle hair that grows shortly after *The Big Chop* as "scab hair". The scab phase can last anywhere from two to eighteen months. But as your mane starts to heal, it will soon start to feel soft and moisturized once again.

I just went natural six months ago. Whenever I put products on my hair, they just sit there. What products can I use to give my hair some moisture and shine?

Don't forget: less is more. Try to keep your product usage to a minimum. Natural oils, like sunflower, jojoba, and sweet almond oil are light and great for keeping the hair moisturized. Be sure to avoid products that contain lanolin and petroleum, which can leave the hair looking dull and feeling coated. Giving yourself a good clarifying treatment once a month to eliminate product buildup should also help your situation to improve. And keep in mind that kinky hair, due to its shape, doesn't shine -- but it does have a natural sheen. If you continue having trouble, check out the Salon Directory to locate a natural hair care expert in your area who can provide you with further information.

Now that I am natural, do I need to trim my ends?

YES! Even though you're natural, you still need to get your ends clipped. It's a good idea to trim your hair every three to four months to avoid split ends and minimize knots and tangles. Keeping your ends trimmed will also help your hair to look thick and healthy. *Note:* I would highly recommend having your ends trimmed by a professional. When it comes to keeping your hair in tiptop shape, it's always great to have a second opinion.

In some parts of my head, my hair is loose and spirally, while in other parts it's tight and kinky. What advice can you offer for dealing with these two different textures?

It's fairly common to have different textures throughout your hair. My best advice would be to accept the textures for what they are and don't fight against them…embrace them. I used to get frustrated when my twist outs would come out fuzzy in the back and curly everywhere else. Now, I just go with the flow, smile, and accept the compliments when they come my way.

Is it okay to press my hair?

The only time I wear my hair pressed is when I get my ends trimmed. But even this small amount of heat has sometimes left me with a few straight strands here and there. Plus, the style only lasts for two three days before I need to pull my hair back into a ponytail or bun. If you're looking to wear your hair straight for a special occasion, consider wearing a wig or getting a sew-in-weave. Wigs and weaves are great alternatives to flat ironing the hair, giving you versatility without the damage. If you choose to get a press, make sure you find someone who is knowledgeable about natural hair and can achieve good results -- without causing heat damage.

What is Shea butter? Where can I buy it?

Shea butter comes from the shea nut of the Shea-Karite tree, which has its origins in West Africa. Westerners have recently discovered the unique healing properties of shea butter -- but this natural ingredient has been a mainstay in African culture since ancient times. It's very rich, making it great for eliminating dry scalp, breakage, and split ends. The moisturizing and smoothing properties of shea butter have also been used to treat dry skin, diaper rash, sunburn, eczema, and minor burns. Shea butter is available in its pure form online at www.fromnaturewithlove.com and at your local health store or African import market. If you purchase products that contain less than 100% shea butter, read the label to make sure it's among the first few ingredients listed. If it isn't, the product probably only contains trace amounts and will not have the desired effect.

My hair is 6" long -- but it looks half as long. What can I do to fix this problem?

Shrinkage is just a normal part of being natural. I tell everyone this: it is always easier to work with your natural texture, rather than against it. You can wear two strand twists for a couple of days to help stretch out the curls and then try to unravel them for a nice twist out or a chunky 'fro. Some naturals also use a technique known as banding to make their hair look longer. All you need to do is part your hair in six to eight sections and wrap soft ponytail holders down the shaft of each section. If you sleep with your hair this way, you can take it down in the morning and VOILA -- your hair shows more length. Finally, blow-drying and flat ironing your hair will help it to show its true length. But, I can't stress enough, that hair straightening can be damaging if done too frequently.

I'm in the midst of transitioning and have a lot of questions? Where can I go for support?

Two of the best websites online where you can find more information about caring for your natural hair are www.thankgodimnatural.com and www.nappturality.com. You should also check out www.motowngirl.com if you're looking for photos of what you can expect during your transition.

I wash my hair once a week and use a moisturizing pomade everyday, but my hair still feels dry and brittle. Help!!!

There are several things that may be causing this problem. First off, your hair may start to feel dry and brittle if you're using too many products or too much of the same product. Instead of being absorbed by the hair, the product(s) will start to build-up and coat the hair shaft. Second, stay away from products with a high lanolin or petroleum content and stick to natural oils, which are light and easy for the hair to absorb. Third, many shampoos contain harsh detergents, which can strip the hair of its natural oils. Consider switching to a milder shampoo or try washing your hair with conditioner instead (*no-pooing*) for a few weeks and see if you notice any improvement.

I read somewhere that it is good to wash your hair with apple cider vinegar. Is this true?

An apple-cider vinegar (ACV) rinse is like an all-natural, clarifying treatment that helps to remove product buildup and residue from the hair and scalp. Many naturals report that doing an ACV rinse leaves their hair feeling soft and shiny. Check out Chapter 15 -- Making Products at Home -- for an ACV recipe and other homemade hair treatments that will soon have your mane looking soft and luxurious.

Styles

I am starting to see more natural hairstyles in black magazines. But no matter how hard I try, I can never get my hair to look like the models. What am I doing wrong?

240

I wish I could tell you that you were doing something wrong -- but in reality, you're probably not. The truth is that many of these models are wearing wigs, weaves, and extensions. However, there is no need to feel discouraged. Your hair stylist should be able to work with your texture and length to help you create a similar look using your own natural hair. Also, explore my website and check out the step by step instructions on how to achieve these styles at home or purchase a copy of Nedjetti's No Extensions Hair DVD available at www.naturalhairdvd.com for live demonstrations of natural hair styles being created on models without extensions.

I'm getting married next month. What natural styles do you think look good under a wedding veil?

First of all, congratulations and best wishes for a long and happy marriage! Now, when it comes to natural hair, you have plenty of styling options. Although I love my twist-outs, this style can be somewhat unpredictable depending on the weather conditions. I say your best bet would be to go with two strand twists, comb coils, or a straw set. These are all great choices for just about any special occasion and will hold up well in most climates.

Locks

What are locks?

Locks are matted strands of hair which form when the hair is allowed to grow naturally over long periods of time. The expression *"dreadlocks"* originated in Jamaica as a derogatory term used to describe the hairstyle frequently worn by Rastafarians. Although Bob Marley is often credited with popularizing this hairstyle, its origins can be traced all the way back to ancient Egypt and is even found in many passages throughout the Bible. This beautiful hairstyle can be worn as an expression of spirituality, cultural heritage, and politcal perspective -- or merely as a fresh, fashion statement.

What are Sisterlocks?

Sisterlocks are super thin locks created using a crochet like instrument. Depending on their size, the average individual with this hairstyle has between 350-450 Sisterlocks. In comparison, an individual with traditional locks typically has between 100-150 locks. For more information about Sisterlocks or to locate a Sisterlocks consultant in your area, visit www.sisterlocks.com

How do I start locks?

Locks can be started using braids, two strand twists, comb coils, palm rolls or lock extensions. Alternatively, kinky hair will lock naturally if it is allowed to grow without any manipulation (e.g. combing, brushing, trimming, etc.) over time. For more information about each method, check out Chapter 9 – Get Lock'd Up.

How much hair do I need to start locks?

You need at least two inches of natural hair to start regular locks -- but you can start Sisterlocks with one-half inch of either relaxed or natural hair.

I want locks, but I'm scared that my styling options will be limited.

With locks, your styling options are quite endless. You can twists your locks for a crinkly look, wear them pinned up in a classy up-do, highlight them for a different look, or even cut and layer your locks for a whole new style. Check out Thierry Baptiste's website at www.thierrybaptiste.com for the latest trends in styling and coloring your locks. Your styling options are only as limited as your creativity and imagination.

Should I start my locks myself or have them professionally done?

Although many people are capable of maintaining beautiful locks at home, I would highly recommend having your locks started professionally. A professional locktician can help you achieve locks that are uniform in shape and size, which will increase your styling options in the long run and provide your hair with a strong foundation as it grows longer.

Will my hair grow longer with locks?

We have all seen people with waist-length locks. But in actuality, the hair strands are never this long. Locks are simply strands of shed hair or regular length matted together.

Can I wash my hair if I have locks?

Yes -- but most lockticians generally advise their clients with starter locks to avoid washing their hair the first three weeks to give their locks the chance to settle. During this time, an antiseptic cleanser, like Sea Breeze, or a light herbal hair mist should be used to cleanse the scalp. If you lead an active life or have a scalp condition and need to wash your locks sooner, cover your hair with a nylon stocking and shampoo your hair as usual. The worst thing that can happen is that some of your locks will begin to unravel -- but they can easily be re-twisted. Once your hair starts to lock, then it's safe to wash your hair at least once a month or more frequently, as you see fit.

How do I maintain my locks?

Again, you should be washing and conditioning your locks at least once a week. When it comes to re-twisting your locks, use an alcohol free styling product (which has its own holding properties) to help your new growth matte. But be careful not to over twist your locks. *Remember:* the less you manipulate your hair the better. Over-twisting can also cause your locks to become thin or break off. For more detailed information on caring and maintaining for your locks, check out Chapter 9 - Get Lock'd Up.

What if I decide I don't want locks anymore? Do I have to cut off all of my hair?

Many people don't realize until long after they have cut off their locks that it's possible to take down their locks and save their hair. Although this long and tedious process requires a great deal of patience, it can be done using a cream conditioner and a sharp instrument to pick apart the lock. Many salons also offer this service -- but you should expect to pay between $250-$500.

Color

Will my color come out the same shade as the picture on the box?

In most cases, it won't. The outcome will depend on your natural hair color, residue left from previous coloring, your last deep conditioner, and other factors. If you have a specific color in mind, you might be better off going to a salon and having your color done professionally. More often than not, it's worth spending the extra $30 upfront to avoid having to pay $75 (or more) later to have the color corrected.

I dyed my hair auburn six months ago but would now like to color it back to black. Can I just dye over it?

Yes, but remember the famous words, once you go black you never go back! Unless you're absolutely sure that you'll like the new color, consider having a professional perform this service in order to avoid over processing your hair.

I just colored my hair and don't like the result. How long do I have to wait before I recolor?

In most instances, color correction can be performed the same day. However, this is a job for a professional. A color expert, who specializes in corrective work, should be able to save your hair from further damage and treat the mishap using safe and gentle products. Remember, out-of-the-box products are typically not sophisticated enough to solve a coloring mishap. So, your best bet is to leave it to the pros.

234

How long should I leave my color on for?

Never leave your color on for longer than the amount of time listed on the instructions. *Note:* it is important to read the instructions each and every time your color your hair. Your favorite brand may have changed its formula and different brands have different time requirements. Again, you'll want to minimize your exposure to color, since these chemicals found in hair dyes can be harmful to your health.

How do I keep my color from fading?

To prevent premature fading, use a color treated shampoo like Aveda's Color Conserve Shampoo. Using a deep conditioner at least three days before coloring your hair will also give you better results. Hair that is deep-conditioned will absorb color better, causing the color to last longer. It's also a good idea to avoid chlorine and over-exposure to the sun. For more tips on keeping your color rich and vibrant, check out Chapter 10 - Color Me Natural.

Is it safe to dye my hair, if I am almost completely gray?

Usually it is – but gray hair can be extremely resistant to hair color. For maximum coverage, leave the hair dye on for the full amount of time listed on the instructions and sit under the dryer with a plastic cap covering your head.

Is it safe to dye my hair if I am pregnant?

The jury is still out on this issue. Although it is believed that small amounts of hair dye are absorbed into the bloodstream, the effects these chemicals have on your unborn child remain largely unknown. Dr. Shari Brasner, an obstetrician at Mount Sinai Medical Center in New York City and the author of *Advice From a Pregnant Obstetrician*, advises her patients to be "conservative in the critical first ten weeks of pregnancy," while some doctors discourage the use of chemial hair services for the entire duration of the pregnancy. To be safe, you should speak with your Ob-Gyn before having any type of chemical service performed.

235

Hair Loss

What causes hair loss?

For many women, the day-to-day stress -- caused by balancing the responsibilities of work and family -- is a major cause of hair loss. Genetics may also be a factor. But, in most instances, hair loss can be traced back to unhealthy styling practices and/or changes in hormone levels. Excessive heat from blow-drying, curling, or pressing the hair will always eventually take its toll on even the healthiest tresses. Fluctuations in your hormones caused by pregnancy, menopause, stress, chemotherapy, and poor nutrition can also trigger hair loss. The good news is that most cases of hair loss can be treated with medication, vitamins, or hair replacement surgery -- or camouflaged with hair extensions, wigs, or a change in hairstyle.

Is Rogaine safe to use? What are its side effects?

Rogaine is the first FDA-approved product proven to re-grow hair and to stop hair loss. This product is safe for use by women and is now available without a prescription. Some users, however, experience scalp irritation, redness, and dandruff -- but these side effects can be treated with an over-the -counter medicated shampoo like Nizoral or Neutrogena T-Gel. Due to its alcohol content, some individuals may develop a rash. Over-use of this product may also result in dizziness, fever, or increase the heart rate. However, such occurrences are rare with proper usage.

Why won't my hair grow past a certain length?

Hair grows at the rate of a one-quarter to one-half inch each month, depending on your genetic make up. Rather than obsessing about growing your hair long, shift your focus to maintaing healthy hair. Remember, you always have more styling options when your hair is short and healthy versus when it's long and damaged. In the meantime, eating a healthy diet, getting plenty of rest, drinking lots of water, and limiting your use of blow dryers and flat irons are just a few things you can do to keep your hair looking healthy and beautiful.

Do women with natural hair suffer from hair loss?

Absolutely!! Although natural hair is healthier hair, women who are natural still suffer from split ends, breakage, hair thinning, and hair loss. This is why it is essential to master the fundamentals of good hair care.

How effective are hair transplants?

Hair transplants have come a long way in recent years due to breakthroughs in technology and advancements in surgical techniques. This highly sophisticated yet relatively simple procedure offers remarkably natural results for women who suffer from balding or thinning hair. The quality of hair restoration specialists vary widely, so it is important to perform extensive research to ensure your physician is up to date on the latest techniques. For more information about hair transplant surgery -- or to locate a certified physician in your area -- visit www.hairtransplantnetwork.com.

I am interested in learning more about hair transplants. Where should I go to get more information?

For more information about hair transplants, visit www.hairtranspla ntmagazine.com. This website features over 500 hair transplant photos, profiles of some of the nation's most respected hair transplant surgeons, and FAQ's about hair transplants -- as well as a message board where you can discuss your questions and concerns with actual doctors and other patients.

247

*Natural
Hair Glossary*

A

ACV Rinse – For years, health experts have touted the benefits of apple cider vinegar (abbreviated ACV) for promoting healthy, shiny hair. When used as a final rinse, apple cider vinegar helps to seal the hair's cuticle and remove product build-up left by commercial shampoos.

Afro – A natural style in which the hair surrounds the head like a halo or a cloud. Feeling divine? Wear one of these rockin' do's!

Alicia Keys – Grammy award winning artist known for her musical talents as well her freshly cornrowed styles. This bi-racial beauty has scored major hits with such songs as "*Diary*", "*You Don't Know My Name*", and "*If I Ain't Got You*" – and always looks fabulous with her own unique style.

Aloe Vera – A soft gel-like substance produced by the leaves of the Aloe plant. This natural moisturizer is frequently used in shampoos and pomades to help restore or maintain a healthy moisture balance. Aloe is also beyond compare for its soothing properties and can help to relieve dry and itchy scalp. You can buy it as a beauty product or enjoy the interesting looking and easy to grow plant in a sunny window. Just keep it watered and enjoy an endless supply of pure, organic Aloe Vera. When you need some, just break a leaf off the plant and squeeze.

Alopecia – The medical term for hair loss.

B

BAA – An acronym for Big Ass Afro. Check out the 1970s flick Foxy Brown and see gun-toting Pam Grier bring her foes to their knees with this sexy style.

Badu – See Erykah Badu.

Banding – A technique used during slavery and by some modern naturals that involves wrapping thread or pieces of a cloth around a section of hair to make it stretch and appear longer.

Bantu Knots – Hairstyle of South African origin consisting of many small buns. Using braids or twists, hair is wound repeatedly around itself to form small bumps or buns. The style is also commonly referred to as China Bumps or Nubian Knots.

Big Chop – (Not to be confused with the Lorena Bobbitt!) The glorious moment when an individual cuts off all of their relaxed ends and wears their hair completely natural. As in, "After transitioning for ten months, I decided to do *The Big Chop*." If it sounds terrifying, don't let it freak you out. It can be terrifically liberating. If you are feeling stressed, call on your natural buddy for support and encouragement.

Blow Out – A style where the hair is blow-dried and left as is or flat ironed for a silky smooth finish.

Build-up – The residue that develops on your hair and scalp from the use of too many hair products and styling aids.

C

Carcinogen – These are any substances or agents known to cause cancer. Talk about dying to look beautiful.

Cholesterol – Too much of this stuff can cause real problems for your heart's health -- but this ingredient can also be found in hair conditioners that give luster, body and softness to dry brittle hair.

Chunky Afro – An Afro that is worn with minimal manipulation or created by braiding the hair, unraveling it, and finger combing it for added texture and volume.

Claire Huxtable – the successful attorney and wife of Bill Cosby's character, Cliff Huxtable -- on the smash hit television sitcom *The Cosby Show*. Played by actress Phylicia Rashad.

Clarifying Treatment – A product, usually a shampoo, that removes residue and traces of mineral deposits left on the hair and scalp from frequent use of hair styling aids. Think of it as a refresher for your tresses.

Comb Twist – A locking technique, where sections of the hair are twisted in a spiral motion using the teeth of a rat-tail comb, to produce a spiral coil.

Combination Hair – Hair that is oily at the scalp and dry at the ends.

Conditioner – A product most commonly used after shampooing the hair to restore moisture and improve detangling and manageability.

Conditioner Washes – See No-Poo.

Cool Tones – When coloring your hair, you'll want to choose shades that compliment your eye color and skin tone. In general, your skin tone is cool if your natural hair color is bluish-black, dark brown, or golden brown.

Cornrows – A traditional African hairstyle where the hair is plaited close to the scalp to produce a continuous raised row.

2H

Curl Definition – An indicator of the precision of the hair's curl pattern (e.g. some products promise to cut down on frizz and improve "curl definition").

Cuticle – Structure that forms the outermost layer of the hair shaft. The condition of the hair is generally determined by the health of the cuticle.

Cortex – This structure is composed of rope-like fibers and forms the middle layer of the hair shaft. The strength, elasticity, growth pattern, width, texture, and color of the hair are determined by the composition of the cortex.

D

Dandruff - A condition caused by excessive shedding of dead skin cells from the scalp, which may result in visible white flakes on the head, neck and shoulders (and make it embarssing to wear black).

Deep Conditioner – An intense conditioning treatment that restores moisture, increases elasticity, and imparts shine to your strands. This product can also help to repair damage caused by styling manipulation, chemical treatments, coloring, heat styling, and environmental pollution.

Denman – A styling brush with plastic bristles set in an anti-static rubber cushion. The D3 is one of my favorite styling tools and is great for detangling naturally curly hair when wet.

Demi-Permanent Hair Color – See Semi-Permanent Hair Color.

Dilute – To add water with the purpose of thinning or reducing the concentration of a mixture.

Double Boiler (also called a bain-marie) – A technique used by soap-makers and hobbyists to warm/melt ingredients to a fixed temperature. A double boiler generally consists of two pans -- a large container filled with water and a smaller container filled with the ingredients to be heated. The smaller container is then placed inside the larger container -- and the larger container is heated.

Dreadlocks – Initially a derogatory term that originated in Jamaica -- used to describe the hairstyle worn by members of the Rastafari sect.

E

Erykah Badu - Neo-soul singer known for her trademark head-wraps -- as well as major hits like *"Tyrone", "Next Life Time", Bag Lady", and "On and On".*

Essential Oils - The aromatic compounds extracted from the seeds, roots, bark, and berries of plants used in perfumes, cosmetics, incense, and aromatherapy products. Because of their natual origins, essential oils tend to be more expensive then fragrance oils, which are often synthetically derived. The aroma they provide is clear, clean, and pure. Ahhh.

F

Family Ties – Popular 1980s sitcom starring Michael J. Fox as Alex P. Keaton -- the conservative business-driven (and Republican) son of liberal parents Meredith Baxter-Birney and Michael Gross.

FDA – The United States Food and Drug Administration, abbreviated FDA, is the government agency responsible for the oversight and regulation of food, drug and cosmetic preparations.

Fine Hair - A hair shaft with a small diameter.

Finger Comb – A technique where one uses the fingers instead of a comb to style the hair. This practice offers a gentle alternative to manipulating the hair with typical styling utensils.

Finger Parting - A technique, where one uses the fingers instead of a comb to part the hair. This practice offers a gentle alternative to manipulating the hair with regular styling utensils.

Finger Twist – A technique, where small sections of hair are rolled around the fingers to produce a finger-size spiral curl.

Flat Twists – A hairstyle similar to cornrows where the hair is twisted instead of braided flat against the scalp to produce a continuous raised row.

Floetry – English Neo-soul duo best known for their freeform hairstyles and soulful hits like *"It's Getting Late"*, *"Floetic"*, and *"Say Yes."*

Follicle – See Hair Follicle.

Fragrance Oils – Synthetically derived compounds used to give flavor or aroma to perfume, cosmetics, and food preparation. Fragrance oils, however, do not possess the natural properties of essential oils since they are not extracted from botanical (plant) ingredients.

Freeform locks – See Organic Locks.

G

GerryLocks – A locking technique developed by Gerry Mayo, owner of Endless Creations of You Salon, Upper Darby, PA to give fullness to thinning locks and to replace damaged and/or broken locks.

Glycerin – Derived from palm oil, glycerin is a natural humectant and conditioning agent that helps your hair to attract and retain moisture. This ingredient is easily absorbed by the hair shaft and is frequently used in shampoos and conditioners to increase their moisturizing properties.

Growing Pains – Popular 1980s sitcom starring Kirk Cameron and Tracey Gold (and a pre-"Titanic" Leonardo DiCaprio in its final season) that dealt with the issues facing a family when a stay at home mother returns to work as a television reporter.

Guanidine Hydroxide Relaxer – See No-lye Relaxer.

H

Hair Follicle – A tiny sac-like structure that lies below the surface of the skin from which the hair shaft grows.

Hair Shaft – Dead strands of protein that emerge from the hair follicle, which are visible above the scalp.

Hand In Fro Disease – A condition characterized by the constant urge to touch one's own natural hair. Not uncommon in black, white, Hispanic, or Asian men in close proximity to beautiful black women with puffs, locks, and two strand twists.

Henna – An all-natural alternative to synthetic hair dyes, which gives the hair a deep auburn or burgundy tint.

Humectant – an ingredient that attracts moisture.

I

INCI – The International Nomenclature of Cosmetic Ingredients, abbreviated INCI, is an international system developed by the American Cosmetic, Toiletry, and Fragrance Association used to name and identity the ingredients on cosmetic packaging.

Isabella Broekhuizen – Aspiring model from the Netherlands, whose modeling career was ended prematurely when chemical burns caused by a relaxer left her bald and disfigured.

J

Jill Scott – Beautiful soul songstress who has won fans over with her amazing voice, as well, as her signature chunky 'fro. Famous for hits like *"Getting in the Way"*, *"Long Walk"*, and *"He Loves Me"*.

Jojoba Oil – An oil extracted from the seeds of the desert shrub simondsia chinesis, which closely resembles the natural sebum produced by the scalp. This emollient restores shine and manageability to natural hair, without causing product build-up or leaving a sticky residue.

K

Keratin – A strong, insoluble protein substance that is the primary structural component of hair and nails.

L

Lauryn Hill – Former member of the rap group the Fugees, famous for her trendsetting locks and soulful vocals. Major hits include *"Killing Me Softly"*, *"That Thing (Doo Wop)"* and *"Lost Ones"*. Lauryn, where have you been lately? We miss you!

Lanolin – A cheap, greasy substance derived from sheep -- widely used in styling pomades formulated for black hair that offers no real moisturizing benefits. Good for the flock's locks but not our tresses, thanks.

Leave-in Conditioner – A conditioner that does not need to be rinsed out after it is applied to the hair.

Lecithin – A wax like substance derived from soybeans, which acts as an emulsifier (prevents oil and water based ingredient from separating) and thickening agent in cosmetic preparations.

Lo-poo – A hair care maintenance routine that consists mainly of conditioner washes, but includes using a regular shampoo on occasion (once every two to three weeks).

Locks – Matted strands of hair which form when the hair is allowed to grow naturally over long periods of time

Locktician – A hair stylist who cares for and maintains locks.

LOIS System – A system for classifying hair type developed by http://ourhair.net, which incorporates most African-American hair types and eliminates the hierarchal concept of "good hair" and "bad hair".

M

Mariah Carey – American pop star famous for her gorgeous wavy tresses and chart topping hits, such as *"Vision of Love"*, *"Shake It Off"*, and *"We Belong Together"*.

Medulla – The innermost layer of the hair shaft, which is composed almost entirely of soft protein.

Melanin – A chemical substance found in humans, which gives the hair and skin its natural color/pigment.

Microbraids – A style that is achieved by braiding the hair into extremely small braids using human or synthetic hair.

MotownGirl – A fellow Detroiter who has launched a popular website dedicated to helping people learn how to style and care for their natural hair at home. Filled with product reviews, homemade hair care recipes, and step by-step styling instructions, www.motowngirl.com should be on your list of top places to visit when going natural.

N

Nappturality – An online community which features chat rooms, photo galleries, and articles of interest to women who are natural or in the process of transitioning. Check out this popular website at www.nappturality.com.

Natural – Noun used to refer to a person with natural hair.

Natural Buddy – Your personal 411/911 who offers information, guidance and support for the natural journey. In return, you of course, provide the same for them as needed. This is the person you call when you're facing critical moments and making major hair decisions, like when it's time to do *The Big Chop* or when your stylist tries to convince you to return to the Dark Side. You and your natural buddy must stay strong and support each other.

Natural Hair – Hair that is not chemically relaxed or texturized.

No-lye Relaxer –There are three types of hair relaxers: sodium hydroxide, guanidine hydroxide, and ammonium thioglycolate. Guanidine hydroxide relaxers are commonly referred to as "no-lye" relaxers and tend to be less damaging than sodium hydroxide relaxers. These products, however, may still cause harm to the hair and should always be applied by a trained professional.

No-Poo – A way to wash the hair without shampoo. In her book *"Curly Girl"*, Lorraine Massey recommends that women with curly hair wash their hair only with conditioner for added shine and softness. Hence the name, No-Poo. (Sounds silly -- like a toilet training command, I know, but it's really a good thing for the hair!)

Non-Hodgkin's Lymphoma – Cancer of the lymphatic system - the body's blood-filtering tissues that help to fight infection and disease. According to the American Cancer Association, women who use dark hair dye for two decades or more are four times more likely to develop this condition.

Normal Hair – Hair that is neither oily nor dry.

O

Organic – Word used to describe a product that contains all natural ingredients and no synthetic or artificial additives. At this time, there is no official, legal definition of this term.

Organic Locks – Locks which are started and maintained completely without manipulation. Hair is washed and left alone (e.g. no combing, brushing, trimming, etc.). Also, known as Freeform locks.

P

Panthenol or Pro Vitamin B – An ingredient used in hair care products to impart sheen, improve manageability, and replenish moisture. Panthenol or Pro Vitamin B has also been shown to increase the strength and thickness of hair, making it far more resistant to breakage, split ends, and damage caused by brushing, blow drying, chemical services, and the environment.

Parabens – A preservative used to extend the shelf life of most cosmetics and personal care products.

Patch Test – A process where a chemical is applied to the skin to determine if it causes an allergic reaction. A patch test is always advisable when working with chemicals, such as color or relaxers. Also, it's a good idea to test an area of skin that's not super visible. So, avoid the face and neck, and go for the wrist instead. This way, if something ugly erupts, you won't have to be bothered with your co-workers asking you silly or embarrassing questions (as you know they would!).

Permanent Hair Color – Products used to color the hair. Unlike semi-permanent dyes, permanent hair color contain high amounts of ammonia and peroxide and do not rinse out when the hair is shampooed.

Petroleum – A cheap, greasy substance widely used in styling pomades formulated for black hair. Unlike natural oils, petroleum offers no real moisturizing benefits and it leaves you smelling like an oil tanker. Mmm, how romantic!

pH – Power of Hydrogen, abbreviated pH, is used to measure the acidity/base levels of a substance. The pH scale ranges from 0 to 14. A pH of 7 means that a substance is neutral. Pure water, for example, has a pH of 7. A pH below 7 means a solution is acidic. A pH above 7 means the solution is basic. The less the pH, the more acidic the solution. Conversely, the greater the pH, the more basic the solution. A typical human hair has a pH of 4.5 to 5.5.

Plopping – A technique used on freshly washed hair to help remove excess moisture and give hair strands curl definition. For best results, bend over from your waist and gather the bulk of your hair near the top of the head and secure with a super absorbent towel. Let hair dry ten to fifteen minutes. Remove the towel, shake down the curls and apply styling gel or spritz for extra hold.

Pomade – A styling aid used to mold or sculpt hair into place.

Ponytail – A hairstyle where the hair is pulled into place and secured with a rubber band, scrunchie, etc. (Remember the famous scrunchie episode on "Sex and the City" and the argument between Carrie and Berger that ensued? Berger learned that no real New Yorker wears a scrunchie in public! But I digress…)

Porosity – The measure of the hair's ability to absorb moisture. The hair's porosity is determined by the condition of the cuticle layer. Hair with low porosity can be difficult to color or relax, because chemicals are not readily absorbed by the hair shaft due to the cuticle being closed. Hair with high porosity readily absorbs moisture, because the cuticle layer is open. Overly porous hair also tends to be dry, because it also releases moisture more frequently.

Preservatives – Ingredient used in food and cosmetic preparations that prevents the growth of bacteria and extends the shelf life of products.

Product Junkie – An individual who purchases excessive amounts of styling products. You know you are one when you go into your local Walgreens or CVS for a pack of gum and end up filling one of those little plastic baskets to the brim with nearly a hundred dollars of cute little bottles and jars of who-knows-what that you know you'll never use more than once.

Protective Hairstyles – Hairstyles that don't require frequent manipulation (e.g. braids, cornrows, bun, etc.).

Propylene Glycol – A humectant commonly found in most shampoos to give a product "glide" or "slip". This chemical is also an active ingredient in anti-freeze, airplane de-icer, and brake and hydraulic fluid.

Protein Reconstructor – An intensive repair treatment, which helps to restore strength, structure, body, shine, and moisture to severely damaged hair.

Puff – Style where the hair is gathered together with a bra-strap headband, pantyhose headband, or scarf and worn loose. Ideal style if the hair is not long enough to be worn in a ponytail or if the wearer would like to reduce tension along the hairline. The term may also refer to an Afro-ponytail hair attachment.

R

Reconstructor – See Protein Reconstructor.

Rogaine – The first FDA-approved product proven to re-grow hair in the crown area and stop hair loss.

S

Scab Hair – The dry brittle hair that grows from the scalp shortly after doing *The Big Chop* is often referred to as scab hair. The scab phase can last anywhere from two to eighteen months, but as your hair follicles start to heal, your strands will begin to feel soft and moisturized again.

Sebaceous Glands – Oil producing glands that secrete a natural conditioner (sebum), which keeps the hair soft and moisturized.

Sebum – The hair's natural oil produced by the sebaceous glands, which keeps your mane soft and moisturized.

Semi-Permanent Color – Hair color which can be used to darken -- but not lighten -- the hair.

Senegalese Twists – A style where the hair is twisted using fiber or human or synthetic hair to extend the length and the time of wear.

Serena Williams – one-half of a tennis dynasty -- and one of the most dominant figures in the history of the sport of women's tennis. As a teen, she was also known for her intricate cornrow styles with white beads on the ends. Younger sister of tennis sensation Venus Williams.

Shea Butter – A natural fat extracted from the fruit of the Karite tree, which grows in Western Africa. Because of its conditioning properties, this natural moisturizer is used in hair dressings and pomades to restore moisture to dry brittle hair, prevent breakage and split ends and promote healthy hair growth.

Shrinkage – Due to its spiral shape, many naturals may experience this condition, where their hair appears shorter in its natural state versus when it is straightened. (Also refers to a funny "Seinfeld" episode with George experiencing shrinkage after going in cold water…)

Sisterlocks – A technique used to create small, thin locks using a crochet-like instrument.

Sodium Lauryl Sulfate (SLS) – A detergent used in most shampoos, shaving creams, and bubble baths for its cleansing effect and foaming properties.

Sodium Hydroxide Relaxer – There are three types of hair relaxers: sodium hydroxide, guanidine hydroxide, and ammonium thioglycolate (thio relaxer). Of the three, sodium hydroxide is the strongest and will typically cause the most damage.

Split Ends – A condition that results when the cuticle is damaged -- causing the hair shaft to feel dry and rough at the ends.

Strand Test – A process where a chemical is applied to a single strand of hair to determine its effect. A strand test is always advisable when working with chemicals, such as color or relaxers.

262

T

Texturizer – A mild relaxer that is left on the hair for a short period of time to loosen the hair's natural curl pattern.

Thick Hair – A hair shaft with a large diameter.

Thio Relaxer – The thio relaxer involves a two-part process, where the hair is straightened first and then set on rods to create a new curl pattern. If you ever had a jheri curl, then your hair was probably treated with a thio relaxer.

Traction Alopecia – Hair loss caused by unhealthy styling products including, but not limited to, tight braids, taut ponytails, sew-in weaves, heat styling, and relaxers.

Transitioning – The time period that lapses between when a woman makes the decision to go natural and does *The Big Chop*.

Transitioner – An individual making the transition from relaxed to natural hair.

Trichologist – An individual who specializes in hair and scalp disorders. Although a trichologist can diagnose hair problems and recommend courses of treatment, this individual may not necessarily be a medical doctor.

TWA – Teeny Weeny Afro, abbreviated TWA, is a short haircut or fade where the hair is cropped close to the scalp.

Two-strand Twists – A hairstyle, achieved by intertwining two separate strands of hair around each other repeatedly. Also known as double-strand twists.

Two-strand Twist Extensions –Two-strand twists created by intertwining synthetic or human hair with the natural hair from root to end for added fullness and length.

253

V

Venus Williams – African-American tennis sensation best known for her 100 miles-per-hour serve and her signature cornrow hair style, with beads on the ends. Older sister of Serena Williams.

Vitamin E – An all-natural, vegetable-derived preservative used in hair and body care products to prevent other oils from turning rancid. This lightweight ingredient is easily absorbed by the hair and is highly regarded for its moisturizing benefits.

Volume – A measuring term used to determine the number of strands per square inch on the scalp. Hair's volume can be described as "thick", "thin", or "fine". So, its possible to be classified as having fine hair that is coarse -- just as you can be classified as having thick hair that is fine.

W

Warm Tones – When coloring your hair, you'll want to choose shades that compliment your eye color and skin tone. Your skin tone is usually warm if your natural hair color is red or brown with reddish highlights.

Wheat Protein – A highly refined, natural protein derived from whole wheat that helps to improve body and impart shine. This protein is often found in shampoos and conditioners formulated for damaged or color treated hair.

Wonder Years – A 1980's Emmy Award-winning television drama whose plot centers on the life of a teenage boy growing up in the late 1960s/early 1970s.

264

255

Additional Resources

Hair-care Books

Basic Care for Naturally Textured Hair: Cultivating Curly, Coily, and Kinky Hair by Diane Carol Bailey

Brown Skin: Dr. Susan Taylor's Prescription for Flawless Skin, Hair, and Nails by Susan C. Taylor

Don't Go Shopping for Hair-Care Products Without Me: Over 4,000 Products Reviewed, Plus the Latest Hair-Care Information by Paula Begoun

Good Hair: For Colored Girls Who've Considered Weaves When the Chemicals Became Too Ruff by Lonnice Brittenun Bonner

Going-natural: How to Fall in Love With Nappy Hair by Mireille Liong-a-kong

Natural Hair-care and Braiding by Diane Carol Bailey

Nice Dreads: Hair-care Basics and Inspiration for Colored Girls Who've Considered Locking Their Hair by Lonice Brittenum Bonner

No Lye: The African American Woman's Guide to Natural Hair-care by Tulani Kinard

Plaited Glory: For Colored Girls Who've Considered Braids, Locks and Twists by Lonnice Brittenum Bonner

The Sisterlocks Book: A Tapestry of Dreams Volume 1 (Sisterlocks Book, Volume 1) by Joanne Cornwell

That Hair Thing: And the Sisterlocks Approach by Joanne Cornwell

Why Are Black Women Losing Their Hair? by Barry L. Fletcher

Arts, History, Politics and Reflections

400 Years Without a Comb: The Untold Story by Willie Morrow

Black Hair: Art, style and Culture by Ima Ebong

Black Folk's Hair: Secrets, Shame & Liberation by Kamau Kenyatt

Blue Veins and Kinky Hair: Naming and Color Consciousness in African America by Obiagele Lake

Dreads by Francesco Mastalia

Hair Matters by Ingrid Banks

Hair Story: Untangling the Roots of Black Hair in America by Ayana Byrd and Lori Tharps

Nappy Journey: The Twisted Road to Natural Hair by Sharon, Ph.D. Chappelle

Nappyisms: Affirmations for Nappy-Headed People and Wannabes! by Linda Mosetta Jones

Tenderheaded: A Comb-Bending Collection of Hair Stories by Pamela Johnson

Children Books

Cornrows by Camille Yarbrough

Happy to Be Nappy (Jump at the Sun) by Bell Hooks

I Love My Hair! by Natasha Anastasia Tarpley

Kids Talk Hair: An Introduction Book for Grown-Ups & Kids by Pamela Ferrell

Kinki Kreations: A Parent's Guide to Natural Black Hair-care for Kids
by Jena Renee Williams

Nappy Hair by Carolivia Herron

Wild, Wild Hair by Nikki Grimes

Magazines

Naturally You Magazine, www.naturallyyoumagazine.com.
The first natural hair-care magazine to hit the Internet AND the stands!
Features beautiful photos of 100% NATURAL styles...no weaves or
extensions!

DVDs

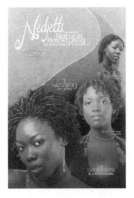

Nedjetti's Natural Hair Styling DVD (Volume 1), www.nedjetti.com

Nautral Hair Websites

www.motowngirl.com

One of the most popular websites online for natural hair-care. Since its
founding in 2001, Motowngirl has been giving her readers an up close
look at hew own natural hair journey. While this site is best known for

its product reviews, it also features information on staying natural, styling tips, and homemade hair-care recipes.

www.afrobella.com

Check out this blog for the latest ruminations on products, fashion, and women in all shades of beautiful. AfroBella definitely keeps it interesting with her commentary on political and social issues and her daily opinions on everything from the meaning of "natural" to her favorite lip-gloss.

www.anappyahairaffair.com

The founder of this website is best known for sponsoring grass roots hair grooming sessions called Hair Days, where black women come together to understand their natural hair-care needs and embrace styles more in keeping with their culture. Check out this site to learn more about Hair Days and find out when the next one is scheduled to take place in your area.

www.brownskin.com

Check out Dr. Susan Taylor's website and find a plethora of resources and information entirely devoted to addressing the special characteristics and needs of brown skin and hair.

www.going-natural.com

Going-natural.com contains inspiring pictures and stories for us by us, a message board to share hair problems, and a nap-shop that offers nappy-friendly products.

www.hairboutique.com

This site offers tips and recommendations on caring for colored treated hair.

www.herspecialhair.com

This website sells e-books (electronic books) designed to assist you with your natural hair-care needs and empower you with the knowledge needed to care for your own hair.

www.longhaircareforum.com

Very active message boards that features tips on transitioning from relaxed to natural hair. Excellent source of information for weaves and wearing natural hair straight.

www.naani.com

This website makes learning about natural hair fun and easy. Click on the hair-"brary", where you'll find online how-to books and articles on everything from the anatomy of hair, treating scalp conditions, and the effects a product has on the pH of your hair.

www.nappturality.com

Whether you're considering going natural or have been natural for years, napptuality has something for women in all stages of their natural journey. One of the most popular sites on the Internet for black women, napptuality features photographs of natural hair, style ideas, hair journals, and articles about care, maintenance, and the politics of natural hair. The natural forums are also a great place to visit if you are looking for answers to your questions and words of encouragement from women that are either in the process of going or are already natural.

www.naturalhairdigest.com

Whether you are starting your hair journey or are a seasoned natural hair wearer, this site has got something to enlighten you! Hair-care, styles, links, articles, and much more.

www.naturallycurly.com

Click on this site to discover how to make the most of your curls. You'll find tips and tricks from experts and reviews of hair-care products. You'll read stories of hair distress that will seem quite familiar -- and you'll be entertained by little snippets of curlydom.

www.OurHair.Net

Website for women with natural, curly, relaxed, kinky, braided, locked, and straight hair. Very active message boards. Be sure to check out the articles on lock maintenance, styling tips, and knowing your hair type.

www.reniece.com/faqs.html

For hair extension reviews and recommendations, check out Weave Specialist Reniece's website.

Lock Websites

www.bigmalik.com

BigMalik.com contains a gold mine of information for individuals thinking about locking. This site traces one man's journey with locks, starting in 2001. The site also features personal journal entries, photos of Malik's hair growth, FAQs, and an online store where can you purchase all of your Big Malik gear.

www.MyDreadLocks.com

No matter what type of hair you have, this lock information site will tell you everything you need to know to get lock'd up. Sign up for the free bi-weekly newsletter online to get lock tips from professional stylists, detailed product reviews, and stylist referrals.

www.howtodread.com

Very active message board, where you can get quick answers to all of your lock questions. Great FAQ Section.

www.knattydread.com

Products designed for maintaining locks.

www.dreadLocks.us

Information on how to start and maintaining locks. FAQs. Photo gallery.

www.dreadlockz.net

Helpful information on starting and maintaining locks. Written in German. Active message boards.

www.dreadLocks.com

Information on starting and maintaining locks. Detailed product reviews. Great facts and rumor section.

www.perfectdreadLocks.com

Perfect place to go if you're looking for detailed product reviews. Information about starting and maintaining locks. Great FAQ Section.

Yahoo Groups

BlackTresses@yahoogroups.com

Active listserv for black women (and men) who have made the decision to stop using heat and chemicals to alter the natural structure of their hair.

LockCity@yahoogroups.com

This discussion group is for anyone who wants information, encouragement, advice and inspirational stories about wearing locks.

Salon Directory

Alaska

Totally Natural Hair Salon - 1569 S. Bragaw Street, Suite 104, Anchorage, Alaska 99508, (907) 338-8186. Anchorage's 1st natural hair salon!

Alabama

Artistic Braids & Naturals - 3102 Greensboro Avenue, Tuscaloosa, AL 35401, (205) 342-3085

Changes Salon & Spa - 1210 32nd Street- North, Birmingham, AL (205) 254-6959

Roots All Natural Styling Salon - 2603 Laverne Drive, Huntsville, AL 35810, (256) 426-9509. *Offering chemical-free, extension free, natural hair-care*

Simply Beautiful – 4000 Marie Avenue, NW # E, Huntsville, AL, (256) 489-2100. *Specializing in braids, cuts, locks and designs.*

Arizona

Cocoa's Braid & Hair Designs - P.O. Box 62152, Phoenix, AZ, 85082,(480) 663-7737. *Specializing locs, natural hair, weaves. Also offering mobile services.*

Hairloks by Arlette - 7000 E. Shea Blvd. Ste.1652 (inside Signature Salon Studios), Scottsdale, AZ 85254, (480) 443-7755. *Specializing in hair care, transitioning from chemical treatments to natural healthy hair. Services include braiding, twisting, locking, lock extensions, hair extensions, the Afro, twist sets and twist outs. Hairlocks also offers classes in the art of natural hair-care and some of the innovative techniques of natural hair care and styling.*

California

Annette's Braids - 4917 S. Western Ave, Los Angeles, CA, (323) 298-0369

Angel Hair Braids - 155 S. Robertson Blvd, Beverly Hills, CA 90211, (310) 659-0064

Cadijah's Loctician Services - Oakland, CA, (510) 681-4112

Flamingo - 5032 Telegraph Ave, Oakland, CA 94609, (510) 658-7223

Hair Today Hair Tomorrow - Adeline Street Lofts, 1131 24th Street loft #118, Oakland, CA 94607, (510) 452-0942, /http://www.hometown.aol.com/cuttinup6951050

I.F.B.A. - Institute of Fine Braidery Arts - 4329 Degnan Blvd., Los Angeles, CA 90008, (323) 299-8994. *Specializing in: straw wraps, lock grooming, twists- single and flat, herbal* *shampoos, corn rows and designer braiding*

Keepers of the Krown - 6519 S. Western Avenue, Los Angeles, CA 90047, (323) 778-5773. *Specializing in locks and lock grooming.*

Margaret's Braids & Weaves - 917 30th St, Sacramento, CA, 95816, (916)203-9923 http://margaretsbraidsandweaves.com

Madu Salon - 300 Divisadero Street, San Francisco, CA 94117, (415) 626-4782, Stylist: Marie France Cesar.

Nappy or Not - 411 E. 18th St., Suite F, Oakland, CA 94606, (510) 835-7838

Oh My Nappy Hair Salon - 805 S. La Brea Ave., Los Angeles, CA 90036, (323) 939-3999

Sisterlocks - San Diego - 858 560 5116, (619) 291-5116, www.sisterlocks.com

Tangles & Locks - 2025 Lake Ave, Altadena, CA, (626)398-9538

The Den Salon - 56556 W. 3rd Street, Los Angeles, CA 90036, (323) 939 6373 Stylists: Dawn Ross

Tying Knots - Inglewood, CA, (310) 677-5987, stayup@sbcglobal.net. *Specializing in Sisterlocks and lock grooming*

Visions Hair Studio - 6926 Federal Blvd., Spring Valley, CA 91977, (619) 460-4652

Colorado

Hair Works -2201 Lafayette St, Denver, CO 80205, (303) 864-1585

Rumors Beauty Salon and Barber Shop - 2350 S. Chambers Road Unit B, Aurora, CO, (720) 748-1400

Connecticut

It's A Gee Thang - 2574 Main St., Hartford, CT 06109, (860) 728-1123 - Rick Nyce and Eunice Smith - Natural stylist and locktician, respectfully

Mahogany's Natural Hair Heaven - 861 Dixwell Avenue, #C, Hamden, CT 06514, (203) 907-3268

Shawne's Mane Attraction - 1325 East Main Street, Waterbury, CT 06702, (203) 754-7666

Twist and Curves – 335 Cottage Grove Ave, Suite D, Bloomfield, CT, 06002, www.twistandcurves.com.(860) 523-4844

Florida

***Natural Trend Setters - 5100 W Commercial Blvd. Lauderhill, FL 33319, (954) 486-1414, www.naturaltrendsetters.com

***Ndigoblue - 269 S. Dixie Hwy, Tampa, FL 33612, (813) 433-6693, www.ndigoblue.com. *Specializing in natural hair styling & care, locks, double strand twist, color, straw sets, etc.*

All Dolled Up - West Oakland Blvd, Sunrise, FL 33441, (954) 428-6678

It's Only Natural - Congress And 45th Street, West Palm Beach, FL, (561) 572-5934, www.HAIRbyJANICE.com. Stylist: Janice Massey

Mandisa Ngozi Braiding Gallery - 1313 N. Gadsden St., Tallahassee, FL, (850) 561-0330 www.mandisa-ngozi.com

Mane-Tain Natural Hair-care - (305) 458-6635. Stylist: Chana. *Specializing in a Convenient Mobile Service. Traveling to meet all your Locking Care Needs. By Appointment only*

Naturally-U Braid Studio - 1241 W. Tharpe Street, Suite C, Tallahassee, FL 32304, (850) 386-8523

Georgia

***Braids, Weaves & Things - 1180 Ralph D. Abernathy, Atlanta, GA 30310, (404) 753-4555. Owner is Taliah Waajid- maker of Black Earth Products

Brown Sugar Studio - 646 Mount Zion Road #B, Jonseboro, GA. 30236, (678)754-6239 *Specializing in Locks and Natural Hair-care*

Contour Images Salon - 4112 Redan Rd., Stone Mountain, GA 30083, (404) 299-9466

Dina Baye Braiding World - 4884 Harrison Pl., Stone Mountain, GA 30088, (404) 299-8912

Natural Beauty Boutique - Duluth, GA, (770) 822-1195 By Appointment Only. Stylist: Wanda

Pure Serenity - Stone Mountain, GA 30088, (678) 643-8197. *Specializing in locks and natural nail care*

Braids Unlimited - 879 Ralph D. Abernathy Blvd. Atlanta, GA 30310, (404) 752-5060

Hawaii

Steven Malani Color Salon - 1600 Ala Moana Blvd, Suite 104, Honolulu, Hawaii, (808) 944-0084

Illinois

***AJES The Salon** - 628 W. Randolph, Chicago, IL, (312) 454-1133

****Time Hair Gallery** – 943 W. Randolph #2W, Chicago, IL (312) 421-5097. Stylist: Kenyon

AMAZON Natural Look Salon - 5548 S. State Street, Chicago, IL, (773) 256-0500

The Abyss Salon – 67 E 16th Street, Chicago, IL 60616, (312) 880-0263

Black Pearl – 7126 Ridge, Chicago, IL, (773) 338-9311

Blyss Full Service Salon – 1703 E. 87th Street, Chicago, IL, (773) 768-8955

Christian Fields Style Bar – 6550 S. Cottage Grove Avenue, Chicago, IL 60637, (773) 288-5627

Desi's Full Service Salon - 2130 West 95th Street, Chicago, IL 60643, (773) 445-8300

DiAnne B. Natural Hair - 1610 West Highland, Chicago, IL 60660, (773) 764-5127, www.DianneBNaturalHair.com. *Specializing in Locks, Loc-Extension, Twist and Sisterlocks/Brotherlocks.*

Freedom Hair Salon – 1518 N. Ashland Avenue, Chicago, IL 60622, (773) 252-4247

Glo On Braids & Natural Hairstyling - (773)643-8299, www.glo-onnaturalhair.com, glo_onbraids@yahoo.com. Stylist: Shavon Akhan

Hair Dare You! - 1459 E. 53rd St., 2nd Fl., Chicago, IL 60615, (866) 384-9386, (773) 288- 0000, contactus @ www.hairdareyou.com.

The Hair Source - 197 Peterson Rd., Libertyville, IL 60048, (847) 573-1993

Kings & Queens Natural Hair Studio - 4519 South Calumet, #1S, Chicago, IL 60653, Jamal West (708) 323-8260, Doug Bradshaw (773) 895-4968. *Specializing in Transitioning ("going natural"), Comb Twist, Loc Maintenance, Loc Repair, Loc Stitch, Double Strand Twist, Crochet Braids, Cornrows, Natural Hair-care/Styles.*

Mane Abstracts - 16 N Morgan Street, Chicago, IL 60607, (312) 666-9999

My First Salon - 1724 East 71st Street, Chicago, IL 60649, (773) 363-1000, www.myfirstsalon.com *Specializing in natural styles for kids.*

Nappy Headz – 4141 North Broadway, Chicago, IL, (773) 549-2664

Red Karma – 3523 S. Indiana Avenue, Chicago, IL, (312) 842-3482

Soul Salon Spa - 4256 S. Cottage Grove, Chicago, IL 60653, (773) 268-3390, www.soulsalonspa.net. *A full service, natural approach to hair, body, skin and nail care; offering Sisterlocks, traditional locks, Afros, braids, and more.*

The Tribesman - 4459 S. Indiana Avenue, Chicago, IL, 60653, (773) 268-6900

Time Hair Gallery – 943 W. Randolph, Chicago, IL, 60607, (312) 421-5097

Toss Hair Salon – 60 E. 13th Street, Chicago, IL 60605, (312) 986-8677

Why Knot Concept Salon - 805 W Randolph Street 203, Chicago, IL 60607, (312) 421-6580

Indiana

*** **Brunette Salon** – Stylist – Thierry Baptiste. http://www.thierrybaptiste.com

Adaru - 6524 N. Carrollton, Indianapolis, IN 46220, (317) 255-2155

269

Louisiana

All Natural Hair Shop - 2273 St. Claude Avenue, New Orleans, LA 70119, (504) 943-0666 email: joalnatural@aol.com

Afritude Hair Braiding Salon, 1418 North Claiborne Ave., Suite 6, New Orleans, LA 70116, (504) 949-9995

Mo Hair Salon - 1345 Gadere Lane, Baton Rouge, LA 70820, (225) 769-2292. Stylist: Joan Louis

Natural Mystiq - 3003 Florida Blvd., Baton Rouge, LA 70802, (225) 343-0067

Nature's Crown - 111 East Airport Avenue, Baton Rouge, LA 70806, (225) 218-8035

Maryland

***Na'Klectic Natural Hair Gallery**- 36 E. 25th Street, Baltimore, MD, 21218 (410) 889-0287, Stylists: Natasha (owner), Jennifer and DiMiriam. www.naklecticnaturalhair.com.

Also offering - natural nail care. Voted #1 Fly Hair Salon of 2006 in Baltimore, MD by the www.flywire.com website and magazine.

***Adunni's Braids and Locks** - 7018 Freeport St., Hyattsville, MD 20784, (301)322-2182

Anel Natural Hair Studio - 10440 Baltimore Ave., Beltsville, MD, 20705, (301) 595 -7108

Artistic Expressions Natural Hair- 6345 Old Branch Ave., Temple Hills, MD, (301) 449 -3737

Changing Faces Hair Boutique - 339 Main Street, Laurel, MD 20707, (301) 497-1500 Stylist: Sherron Algarin

City Styles Braiding Salon - 2204 Hanson Road, Edgewood, MD 21040, (410)679-4548

Conscious Heads Barbershop and Natural Hair Salon - 219 E. 25th St., Baltimore, MD 21218, (410) 889-0100

My Hairitage Natural Hair & Wellness - 7700 Old Branch Ave., Ste A-202, Clinton, MD 20735. (301) 856-0744. *Specializing in holistic hair-care and natural hair and advanced loc techniques workshops.*

Dreadz N' Headz - 1826 Woodlawn Drive Ste. #2, Woodlawn, MD 21207, (410) 298-0660. Stylist: Malaika-Tamu Cooper

Enya's - 13541 Georgia Avenue, Suite 103, Silver Spring, MD, 20906, (301) 933-8111

Jaha Hair Studio - 941 Bonifant Street, Silver Spring, MD, (301) 588-4966

Lovely Locs - 6022 Surrey Sq. Ln., Forestville, MD, 20747 (301) 456-1729

Madam Walker's Braidery - 4015 21ˢᵗ Place, Temple Hills, MD 20748, (301) 505-5313

Natural Blessings - 6039 Red Wolf Pl, Waldorf, MD 20603, (301) 705-8766, www.naturalblessingssalon.com

Natural Locs/Javana or "J" - Baltimore, MD, (443) 744-6131. *Specializing in natural styles, starter locks, maintenance, 2 strands and cornrows.*

Natural-Shapes - Bowie, MD, (202)526-4500. *Specializing in natural hair care, braids, locks, twists, weaves, loc extensions and more...*

Tanglez Natural Hair-care Salon - 4403 Adelle Terrace 1st Fl., Baltimore, MD 21229, (410) 646-0968

The Ultimate Look by Sonya - 10565 Greenbelt Road, Suite B1, Lanham, MD 20706, (240) 481-2180, www.sonyafletcher.com. *Servicing women, men and children. Weaving, braiding, twisting and locking w/excellence. Performing loc extensions, micro locks(alternative to Sisterlocks), the sistah twist collection: Nubian, Afro, Afro curl and loc, Cherokee cornrows, euro*

Salon Directory

locks (strand by strand extensions) and more.

Wisdom Natural Hair-care Salon - 5116 Liberty Heights Ave, Baltimore, MD 21207, (410) 664-1946. Stylist: Tehuti Imhotep

Michigan

***Happy To Be Nappy** - 18957 Livernois, Detroit, MI 48221, (313)340-4247, http://www.happytobenappysalon.com. Stylist: Ewanda Wyndella

Everettes Corn-Rows & Braiding Academy - 16094 E. 8 Mile Rd., Detroit, MI, (313) 527-2884

Locks 4 Life – 10740 Nine Mile Road, Oak Park MI 48237, (248) 545-6100, www.locks4life.com. Stylist: Paulette. *Specializing in Sisterlocks.*

Riccardo's Place - 10333 West 8 Mile Road, Detroit, MI 48221, (313) 342-3300

Minnesota

Malobe Natural Hair Salon - 915 W. Lake St., Minneapolis, MN 55408, (612) 823-8626, www.malobe.com. *Specializing in multi-cultural locks, braids, twists and a host of other natural hairstyles; transitional hair-care (from chemically treated to natural).*

271

V.I.P. Hair & Nail Salon - 1154 Hennepin Ave., Minneapolis, MN 55403, (612) 337-0014.

Missouri

Beauty by Design - 2951 Patterson Rd., Florissant MO 63031, (314) 830-3222

Creative Cuts & Locks Barber & Style - 1723 S New Florissant Rd., Florissant, MO, (314) 524 –4266

Head Turners Hair & Nail Designs - 7524 Florissant Rd., St Louis MO 63121, (314) 381-8880

Jeannine's Hair - 4211 Virginia, Saint Louis, MO 63111, (314) 353-7807

Napps - 6267 Delmar Blvd., Saint Louis, MO, (314) 727 -0312

Natural Hair Reigns N Style - 2944 Derhake Rd., Florissant, MO 63033-3900, (314) 838-9990

Salon Indigo -2319 Woodson Road, St. Louis, MO 63114, (314) 374-7127. www.salonindigo.homestead.com *Specializing in braids, locks, and twists.*

Nevada

The Braid Studio - 2235 E. Flamingo Rd. #302, Las Vegas, NV, (702) 265-6754

New Jersey

***Hair by Nedjetti** - (646) 236 –6726/(973) 923-4817, hair@nedjetti.com, www.nedjetti.com. *Specializing in versatile natural hairstyles without extensions as well as natural hairstyling classes.*

Braids R Us - 301 Irvington Ave., South Orange, NJ 07079, (973) 761-6737. *Specializing in braiding, two-strand twists and locks.*

Creations Between Us Hair Studio, Inc. – 1401 Maple Ave. Hillside, NJ 07112, (973)282-1300

Kukaberrys- (973) 375-2080, Stylist: Keichelle

Mane-Lee-Kinky - 5333 Route 70, Pennsauken, NJ 08110, (856) 66-Curls

New Loc-N-Chop Shop - 170 W Englewood Teaneck, NJ 07666, (201)833-4003

New Mexico

Kamaria Creations - 1501 Mountain Rd NW, Albuquerque NM 87107, (505) 244-9104 www.kamariacreations.com Stylist: Neema Kamaria Hanifa

New York

***Hair by Nedjetti** - (646) 236–6726/(973) 923-4817, hair@nedjetti.com, www.nedjetti.com. *Specializing in versatile natural hairstyles without extensions as well as natural hairstyling classes.*

***Tendrils** - 87 Fort Greene Place, Brooklyn, NY 11217, (718) 875 -3811, www.tendrilshairspa.com

Afrigenix - 220 West 72nd St., New York, NY, (212) 873-0688, www.afrigenix.com

Croom Boutique - 1960 Crotona Ave., Bronx, NY 10457, (718) 299-0643

Khamit Kinks - 327 Gold Street., New York, NY, (718)422-2600, www.khamitkinks.com

MindBodyHair - 3246 White Plains Road Bronx, NY 10467, (718) 324.1037, www.mind-body-hair.com. Stylist: Ebony Hayes. *Specializing in twists, locks, and braids.*

Nubian Kinks - 385 E. 18th Street, Ste 4K, Brooklyn, NY 11226, (718) 703-9550

Thando Kafele (Locktician) - New York, NY, www.thandokafele.com

Turning Heads Beauty Salon & Day Spa - 218 Lenox Ave (Malcolm X blvd), New York, NY 10027, (212) 828-4600, www.turningheadsdayspa.com

North Carolina

***Lockstar Salon -1300 Baxter St, Suite 135, Charlotte, NC 28204, (704)334-6624, www.lockstarsalon.com, Stylist Natasha

Ayana's Glory Locks - Winston-Salem, NC, (336) 765-2090.

Escofhari's Holistic House - 6108 Gateway Dr., Gibsonville NC 27249, (336) 697-9499. Stylist: Robin

God Given Beauty Natural Hair-care Salon - 1554-A Union Road, Suite 104, Gastonia, NC 28054, 704.865.1228, *www.godgivenbeauty.com. Specializing in Sisterlocks, Brotherlocks, starter locks, lock maintenance, braids, twists, cornrows and weaves.*

Schatzi's Design Gallery & Day Spa - 258 W. Millbrook Rd., Raleigh, NC 27609, (919) 844-1933

Natural Roots by Jey - Salon 2001 at 2200 E Millbrook Rd, Raleigh, NC, (919) 308-0262, www.naturalrootsbyjey.com

Taji's Natural Hair Styling - The Avenue Hair Salon, 5300 Atlantic Avenue Suite 103, Raleigh, NC, (919) 332-3021

A Touch of Ambiance -1377 S.E. Maynard, Suite 204, Cary, NC 27511, (919) 469-1414

"Deeply Rooted" a Naturally Rooted Hair-care Studio -2320 Ashley Road, Charlotte, NC 28208, (704) 562-8220. Stylist: Neressia Ross. *Specializing in starter locks, lock maintenance and loc styling.*

Ohio

The Loc Shoppe - 3700 Avalon, Shaker Heights, OH, (216) 921-5410

DJ's Image Beauty Salon - 500 Ross Ave., Cincinnati, OH 45217, (513) 641-3333

Salon Favor - 7370-G Kingsgate Way, West Chester, OH 45069, (513) 779-2147

Pennsylvania

***Duafe Holistic Hair-care**, 2947 W. Girard Avenue, Philadelphia, PA 19130, (215) 232-6850. Stylist/owner: Syreeta Scott A-list roster of clients include Jill Scott, Kindred and Floetry.

Au Naturale - E Chelten ., Philadelphia, PA, (215) 848 -7848

Brownstone Natural Hair & Barber Studio - 1729 South Street, Philadelphia, PA 19146, (215) 545-2555, www.brownstonenaturalhair.com. *Specializing in natural hair-care, locks, double strand Twist, human hair strand-by-strand lock extensions and barbering.*

Thanayi Hair Concepts - 313 Market St., Harrisburg, PA, (717) 232 -7656

Xquisite Hair Design - 1000 Easton Rd., Philadelphia, PA 19095, (215)376-0430, www.xquisitehairdesign.com. Stylist: Nykia

Tennessee

Kinky Rootz Natural Hair Salon – 121 21ˢᵗ Avenue N, Suite 209, , Nashville, TN 37210, (615) 579-0995. Stylist/Owner: Kristi D. Dunkley. *Specializing in undetectable loc extensions, cultivating locks, starter locks, lock styling, undetectable cornrows, braids, twists, and unique natural hairstyles.*

Texas

***Uncle Funky's Daughter** - 2428 Times Blvd., Houston, TX 77005, (713) 528-0888, www.unclefunkysdaughter.com - *"Uncle Funky's Daughter is Houston's premiere natural hair salon and funky clothing boutique. Featuring designs from independent artists and natural hair stylists of color, Uncle Funky's Daughter has already been dubbed as the funkiest, hippest 'lil split personality shop in town."*

Akua Master Loctician and Braider - 6167 Ludington, Houston, TX, (713) 726-9596

Back To Naturel - 2613 Dowling St, Houston TX. 77004, (713) 807-7666

Carolyn's Hair Design - 2013 Wells Branch Pkwy 110, Austin, TX 78728, (512) 252-7655 Stylist: Tiffany

Hair Authority - 10767 Eastex Frwy, Houston, TX 77093, (713) 691-0868

The Institute of Ancestral Braiding - 2642 S. Beckley, Dallas, TX, (214) 946-1460

The Institute of Ancestral Braiding - 17290 Preston Rd. #104, Dallas, TX, (214) 769-6879

Knappi by Nature Lock Shoppe - 4704 Griggs, Houston, TX, (713) 440-8000

Natural Resources - 4715 LaBranch St., Houston, TX, (713) 528-7102

Nubian Xpressions - 6208 Cullen, Houston, TX, 77004-6540, (832) 881-2124

Soul Sister Natural Haircare - 1716 Rosewood, Houston, TX 77004, (713) 521-7685, www.thesoulsister.com

Virginia

Black Butterflies – 3356 Western Branch, Suite E, Chesapeake, VA. (757) 638-2999. Owners/Stylists: Domminique and Vinnes.

BRAIDS & DREADS, 424 N 2nd Street, Richmond, VA, 23219 (804) 278-9114, www.braid-designer.com

Natural Beauty Natural Hair-care Salon - 4857-B Finlay Street, Richmond VA 23231, (804)222-2424, www.Naturalspabeauty.com

Naturally Yours Beauty Salon - Chesterfield Meadows Shopping Center, 6435 Chesterfield Dr., Chester, VA 23832, (804) 778-4861. *Specializing in locks, twists, and braids.*

Shear Elegance Salon - 6535 Auburn Dr., Virginia Beach, VA 23464, (757) 413 9800. Stylist: Contact: Jerry L. Rogers

275

Washington

Anointed Hands Hair Salon/Beauty Supply - 2512 6th St., Bremerton, WA 98312-3922, (360) 782-2409

Gorgeous Braids - 2301 South Jackson, Seattle, WA 98144, (206) 720-0349

Rose's & Siga African Hair Braiding - 6301 Rainier Ave S., Seattle, WA 98118, (206) 725-0077, rosesigabraid@netscape.net

Washington, DC

*** **Noire Salon**- 2221 Kearny St, NE, Washington, DC 20019, (202) 526-2057, www.noiredesignconcepts.com

Natural-Shapes - 1923 New York Avenue, NE, Washington, DC 20002, (202) 526-4500 www.natural-shapes.com. *Specializing in natural hair-care, braids, locks, twists, and weaves.*

Oliver Natural Hair Salon - 5225 Connecticut Ave. N.W. Suite 210, Washington, DC (202) 686-9714

Urban Nature Styles - 2802 Georgia Avenue, NW, Washington, DC 20001, (202) 332-2001, www.urbannaturestyles.com

Twist It Sistah - 317 T St., NE, Washington, DC 20002, (202) 832-3157. *Specializing in locks; creation and maintenance.*

Knotty Naturals Natural Hair-care Salon - 2203 14th St., N.W, Washington DC, 20009, (202) 232-4266. *Specializing in locks, twists, cornrows, braids, loc styles, and healthy hair-care*

Wisconsin

New Wave Styling Studio, 4481 N. 76th Street, Milwaukee, WI 53210, (414) 464-7780. Stylist: Angela Carrington. *Specializing in locks.*

Ontario, Canada

***Strictly Roots Natural Hair-care Studio.** - 154 Bathurst St. Toronto, Ontario, M5V 2R3, (416) 757-1024/(888) 777-8391, www.strictlyroots.ca

***Strictly Roots Natural Hair-care Studio.** - 178 Queen St. East, Brampton, Ontario L6V 1B3, (416) 757-1024/(888) 777-8391, www.strictlyroots.ca

United Kingdom

***Morris Roots** - 184 Tooting High Street, London, SW17 0SF, 020 8672 8003, www.morris-roots.com, morris@morris-roots.com

Akos Braid Design - 139 Balham Hill, London, SW12 9DL 020 8675 3288, http://www.akosbraid.com

Back to Eden Natural Hair and Scalp Clinic - 14 Westmoreland Road, Walworth, London, England SE17 2AY, 0171 703 3173

Bold and Natural - 200 High Road, Leytonstone, London, England E11 3HU, 44 20 8221 0524

Cammalocks - (441) 07855 312 421, South Croydon, England, www.cammalocks.co.uk . Stylist: Marie. *Specializing in Sisterlocks.*

Eftal Natural Hair - 53 West Green, London, England N15 5DA, 0208 8094343, *Specializing in locks, loc extensions, cornrow, silky dreads, straw set, single plaits, weave, cut and trim and much more*

From The Root - 284 Lewisham High Street, London, SE13, 020 8690 2330

Purely Natural - 265 High Road, Leytonstone, London, E11 4HH, 020 8221 1030, anastasiachikezie@hotmail.com

Purely Natural Hair & Beauty, 119 The Grove, Suite 2 , Stratford, London England E15 1EN, 0208 221 0 122, www.purelynaturalhair.com, info@purelynaturalhair.com

Sour 2 Sweet - 24 Great Cambridge Road, London, N17 7BU, 0208 880 9224. Stylist: Angela Plummer.

Streetsahead - 112c Brixton Hill, London, England SW2 1AH, 0208 671 3357

International

***Boucles d'Ebene** - Tel : 06 68 51 20 04, Paris, France, reseau@bouclesdebene.com

Hair Police of Amsterdam - 113 kerkstraat, Amsterdam, Germany

Michael's on Main - Main Street, Chilliwack British Columbia, 1604 792 6161

Magic Style Haarflecht-Atelier - Daimlerstr. 75, 74211 Heilbronn/Leingarten Germany, Tel: 07131/576860, Mobil: 0177/6585641, http://traumfrisuren.de, MagicStyle@Traumfris uren.de. *Specializing in braids, corn rows, locks and hair extensions*

Sera's Beauty Supply/Salon - 1AH Estate Diamond, Christiansted, US Virgin Islands 00851, (340) 778-1000

Photo Credits

A Brush With History

Field Workers Library of Congress Historic Archives
Collection - 1862

Article 2 Chicago Defender

Texture and Type

Hair Follicle Foundationz Limited

In the Pursuit of Nappiness

Twist Out Salon: Hair by Nedjetti. Hair: Nedjetti.com
Photographer: Kade Lam.com
Makeup: Susan Kibutu
Model: Lenore Johnson

China Bumps Salon: Hair by Nedjetti. Hair: Nedjetti.com
Photographer: Eric Von Lockhart
www.EricVonLockhart.com
Makeup: Daniel Green
www.DanielGreenOnline.com

Braids Salon: Prosperity Hair and Beauty Salon
Stylist: Lynette "Pinky" Johnson

Straw Set Salon: Hair by Nedjetti. Hair: Nedjetti.com
Photographer: WayneSummerlin.com
Makeup: Chantal Gesse
Jewelry: Masani Designs.com
Model: Andaye

Wrap Photographer: Fabrice Trombert

Weave Model: Felicia Graham

| **Two Strand Twists** | Salon: Essence of Braiding and Weaving |
| | Stylist: Dionne James-Eggleston |

Get Lock'd Up

| **Baby Locks** | Salon: Uncle Funky's Daughter |
| | Stylist: Tonya Reed |

| **Teenage Locks** | Model: Ericka Ratcliff |

Mature Locks	Photographer: Kestonduke.com
	Model: Paige Williams
	Stylist: Karen Timmons
	Salon: Divine Nubian Creations

| **Sister Locks** | Salon: No Lye Salon |
| | Stylist: Farika |

Stylin' & Profilin'

| **Caesar** | Model: Tara Coyt. Tara is a writer, speaker, and the president of Coyt Communications, an award-winning marketing firm located in Atlanta, GA. She is also an author coach and the founder of the GET IT WRITE Author's Circle. |

| **Twistout** | Model: Miyosha Streets |

| **Bantu Knots** | Salon: Masusu Kinks |
| | Stylist: Nicole Watford |

Kinky Twists	Salon: Hair by Nedjetti
	Hair: Nedjetti.com
	Photographer: Kade Lam.com
	Makeup: Susan Kibutu
	Model: Kim Harris

Afro Puff	Photographer: Levi Walker Model: Rhonda Ray
Weave	Salon: Reneice & Company Stylist: Reneice
Locks	Salon: AJES The Salon Stylist: A.J. Johnson Model: Monique
Crinkly Locks	Salon: Jelani's Naturals Stylist: Jelani
Lock Updo	Salon: Jelani's Naturals Stylist: Jelani
Faux Hawk	Salon: Tendrils Hair Spa Stylist: Diane Bailey
Natural Ponytail	Salon: Hair Lift Hair Care Stylist: Nye Taylor Model: Nye Taylor Photographer: Elijah Lindsay
Coiled Locks	Salon: Hair Lift Hair Care Stylist: Nye Taylor Model: Mbali Taylor Photographer: Elijah Lindsay
Blow Out	Salon: AJES The Salon Stylist: A.J. Johnson
Lock Ponytail	Photographer: Kestonduke.com Model: Paige Williams Stylist: Karen Timmons Salon: Divine Nubian Creations
Flexi Rod Set	Salon: CEO Runway Studios Inc. Stylist: Shante Omotosho

281

Sources

A Brush with History

1 Johnson, Pamela. "Crown and Glory." Essence Aug. 2000.

2 White, Shane and Graham White. Stylin': African American Expressive Culture, from Its Beginnings to the Zoot Suit. Ithaca: Cornell University Press, 1999. p. 48.

3 Morrow, Willie L. Four Hundred Years Without a Comb. San Diego: Morrow Unlimited, 1973. p. 62.

4 Herring, Cedric. Skin Deep: How Race and Complexion Matter in the "Color-Blind" Era. Chicago: Inst. Research on Race & Public Policy, 2003. p. 4.

5 Byrd, Ayanna and Lori Tharps. Hair Story: Untangling the Roots of Black Hair in America. New York: St. Martin's Press, 2001. p. 17.

6 Byrd, Ayana D. and Lori L. Tharps. Hair Story: Untangling the Roots of Black Hair in America. New York: St. Martin's Press, 2001. p. 23.

7 Rooks, Noliwe M.. Hair Raising: Beauty, Culture and African-American Women. New Brunswick, NJ: Rutgers University Press, 2000, p. 26.

8 "C. J. Walker, Madame." http://www.madame-cj-walker.com. Last viewed on September 17, 2007.

9 Bundles, A'Lelia. On Her Own Ground: The Life and Times of Madame C.J. Walker. New York: Scribner, 2001. p. 61.

10 Craig, Maxine. "The Decline and Fall of the Conk; or, How to Read a Process." Fashion Theory. Vol. 1, Issue. 4. Dec. 1997: p.399-419.

11 Craig at 403.

12 Craig at 416.

13 "University Bans Certain Hairstyles for Students". http://www.wtopnews.com/?nid=25&sid=676513. Last viewed on September 17, 2007.

14 Lake, Obiagele. Blue Veins and Kinky Hair: Naming and Color Consciousness in African America. Westport, CT: Praeger Publishers, 2003.

283

Relaxers - How Safe Are They?

15 "Black women awarded $4.5 million in hair care suit - class action case against World Rio Corp. for faulty hair straightening product" Jet. January 20, 1997.

16 "Heading Off Hair-Care Disasters: Use Caution With Relaxers and Dyes." http:

//www.cfsan.fda.gov/~dms/fdahdye.html. Last Viewed on April 26, 2007.

[17] "Heading Off Hair-Care Disasters: Use Caution With Relaxers and Dyes." http://www.cfsan.fda.gov/~dms/fdahdye.htmlu. Last Viewed on April 26, 2007.

[18] Harvard School of Public Health Press Release. Smoking Causes Nearly 5 Million Deaths Annually Worldwide. **September 12, 2003.**

[19] "Study Finds Possible Link between Hair Dye and Bladder Cancer." http://www.cancer.org/docroot/NWS/content/NWS_1_1x_Study_Finds_Possible_Link_Between_Hair_Dye_and_Bladder_Cancer_.asp. Last viewed on May 1, 2007. Manuela Gago-Dominguez, M.D., Ph.D., researcher in preventive medicine at the Keck School and USC/Norris Comprehensive Cancer Center, and her colleagues compared 897 patients with bladder cancer who used hair dye, with a similar number of adults without bladder cancer. The researchers found that the women who used permanent hair dye at least once a month were twice as likely as women who did not use permanent hair dye to develop bladder cancer. These results held true whether or not the women smoked. Note, smoking is the greatest risk factor for bladder cancer.

[20] "Effects of Inhalants on the Nervous System." Neuroscience for Kids. http://faculty.washington.edu/chudler/inhale.html. Last viewed September 19, 2007. See also United States Environmental Protection Agency, *Protecting the Health of Nail Salon Workers*, www.epa.gov/dfe/pubs/projects/salon/nailsalonguide.pdf. Last viewed September 19, 2007.

[21] "Effects of Inhalants on the Nervous System." Neuroscience for Kids. http://faculty.washington.edu/chudler/inhale.html. Last viewed September 19, 2007. See also United States Environmental Protection Agency, *Protecting the Health of Nail Salon Workers*, www.epa.gov/dfe/pubs/projects/salon/nailsalonguide.pdf. Last viewed September 19, 2007.

Color Me Natural

[22] "Study Finds Possible Link between Hair Dye and Bladder Cancer." http://www.cancer.org/docroot/NWS/content/NWS_1_1x_Study_Finds_Possible_Link_Between_Hair_Dye_and_Bladder_Cancer_.asp. Last viewed on May 1, 2007. Manuela Gago-Dominguez, M.D., Ph.D., researcher in preventive medicine at the Keck School and USC/Norris Comprehensive Cancer Center, and her colleagues compared 897 patients with bladder cancer who used hair dye, with a similar number of adults without bladder cancer. The researchers found that the women who used permanent hair dye at least once a month were twice as likely as women who did not use permanent hair dye to develop bladder cancer. These results held true whether or

not the women smoked. Note, smoking is the greatest risk factor for bladder cancer.

Natural? Beware!

[23] Chemical Kids — Environmental Toxins and Child Development. http://www.socialworktoday.com/archive/marapr2007p37.shtml. Last viewed on May 7, 2007.

[24] Propylene Glycol." Living Toxin Free – Your Resource for Healthy Living, http://livingtoxinfree.org/Articles/PropyleneGlycol.htm. Last viewed on September 17, 2007.

[25] Dadd, Debra. Home Safe Home. New York: Putnams (1997).

[26] Terhanian, Harry. Warning: What Your Shampoo's Label Won't Tell You..."
Making Scents Magazine, Summer/Fall 1999.

285